The Art of Positive
AFFIRMATIONS
& MANTRAS

Harnessing the Power for Personal Growth and Fulfillment

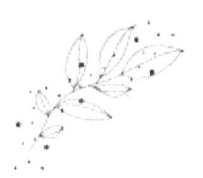

B. M. WOLF

CONTENTS

INTRODUCTION 1

CHAPTER ONE
UNDERSTANDING AFFIRMATIONS AND MANTRAS..................... 3

CHAPTER TWO
CRAFTING POWERFUL AFFIRMATIONS 11

CHAPTER THREE
THE ART OF MANTRAS 22

CHAPTER FOUR
USING AFFIRMATIONS FOR SELF-LOVE, PROSPERITY AND SUCCESS 31

CHAPTER FIVE
EXPLORING SACRED MANTRAS FROM DIFFERENT TRADITIONS 43

CHAPTER SIX
AMPLIFYING RESULTS WITH VISUALIZATION AND MEDITATION 51

CHAPTER SEVEN
AFFIRMATION STATION 61

CHAPTER EIGHT
MINDFUL MANTRA MOMENTS 73

CONCLUSION
EMBRACING THE JOURNEY OF POSITIVE AFFIRMATIONS AND MANTRAS.... 89

BONUS CHAPTER... 92

REFERENCES 98

INTRODUCTION

The Guest House

"This being human is a guest house.
Every morning a new arrival.

A joy, a depression, a meanness,
some momentary awareness comes
As an unexpected visitor.

Welcome and entertain them all!
Even if they're a crowd of sorrows,
who violently sweep your house
empty of its furniture,
still treat each guest honorably.
He may be clearing you out
for some new delight.

The dark thought, the shame, the malice,
meet them at the door laughing,
and invite them in.

Be grateful for whoever comes,
because each has been sent
as a guide from beyond."

— *Rumi - translated by Coleman Barks*

The Guest House is thought-provoking and resonates in the far reaches of my soul. We have all spent time in sorrow, darkness, and pain. When we face that pain head-on and work through it, and accept it, we become better. We become stronger and more wise. Eventually, the pain fades and quietly the laughter with a splash of joy comes back. There have been times in my life when the unexpected visitor has pushed me to look for the light through affirmations and mantras. These treasures have helped to rewire my thinking, gain more prosperity, and find friendships, and love.

Affirmations and mantras are a practice not a light switch. It takes consistency, gratitude, and sheer will. It also takes observations of yourself to find the darkness and negativity inside. Without understanding ourselves, it becomes challenging to change the way our minds work. Inside you will find a thorough understanding of how these positive short phrases can uplift and change your life; and how you can become an active participant as a co-creator of your life instead of letting life happen to you. When I say co-creator, the meaning is to co-create alongside the Divine Universe...and you're driving. The Universe says, "Your wish is my command."

This book is lovingly created by humans from the heart and with a passion to help others raise their own personal vibration and create a life that feels good to live. There are places to journal, pages of affirmations, and mantras to help you find the combination that is right for you. As we grow and change, our affirmations and mantras will grow and change and you can come back to revisit this book over and over again. To recraft new affirmations and try on a new set of mantras.

Our words and thoughts are like magicians' spells, laying the path for our lives to unfold. We can choose a negative narrative widely accepted through common communication, social media, and entertainment, or we can rewire our brains with positive, compassionate, and loving language that sprinkles magic throughout our lives.

Which will you choose?

CHAPTER ONE
UNDERSTANDING AFFIRMATIONS AND MANTRAS

> "The world is a mountain in which your words are
> echoed back to you."
> — *Rumi*

A student of mine, we will call him Roy, was going through addiction treatment earlier in his life. He shared that no matter what kind of meditation he tried, he could never quiet his mind; he lost focus quickly and entered the dreaded rabbit holes. Roy had a lot of anxiety around trying to meditate, even though he knew it would help him. After participating in a meditation class on Kirtan Kriya Yoga and practicing with the mantra of "Saa Taa Naa Maa," he could not believe how fast the 12 minutes of meditation went by. Amazingly, he shared with the group that it was his first time meditating without the distraction of chatter and going down rabbit holes. He found that this was the strongest support in his journey of healing from addiction.

INTRODUCTION TO AFFIRMATIONS AND MANTRAS

To some people, affirmations, and mantras can sound kooky or silly and seem like a futile effort to create change. However, throughout my life, I have used many affirmations and mantras and have found them to be useful tools for creating powerful change within that is reflected in the outer world.

Affirmations are positive words and phrases repeated over and over. They can be placed around your home and office to promote self-belief and motivation along with keeping you on a positive trajectory. Affirmations can be anything from "I can handle this" to "I love my body, my mind, my dreams and my goals." Repeating affirmations is a pattern interrupt for repetitive loops of negative self-talk or reactive emotions that we want to change, often after many failed attempts. Affirmations are effective because they rewire our subconscious mind and create new neural pathways in the brain, which is called neuroplasticity. [1] Having affirmations in your toolbox can truly assist you in gaining control over-reactivity, defensiveness, lack of mentality, and so much more. Neuroscientists know and understand that whatever we impress on our subconscious mind will reflect in our outer world.

What is a mantra, and how is it different from affirmations? In today's modern world, many people will mistake a mantra for an intention or just another positive phrase to say. But it is vastly different. While affirmations are positive statements to rewire our minds, mantras are sounds that emit a specific vibration to harmonize our being with the universe [2]. A mantra is a Sanskrit term that translates to "mind-vehicle". [3] A mantra can be a sound or vibration that harnesses an intention and plants it deep into the fertile soil of our heart and meditation practice. As such, a mantra becomes a vehicle to harness the power of our mind. [4] As we become observers, continue to practice the mantra, and focus on our intentions, we can watch the mantra unfold in our lives.

Mantras are well-known in Hinduism and Buddhism but are now widely accepted in many religious and spiritual traditions. Mantra meditation (MM), also known as primordial sound meditation, has its roots in the Vedic tradition. [5] Primordial sound mantras consist of a personal *bija*, translated to seed. These seed sounds are gifted by a teacher and act as a personal mantra that builds over time. This mantra is more about vibration than meaning. There is no defined meaning. We can't understand this mantra with our minds, as it takes us beyond any preconceived ideas of ourselves. Meditators use mantras to bring greater peace and calm into their lives. Transcendental meditation is a modern school of meditation that uses primordial sound.

There are also *Nakshatra Birthstar Mantras*, which are derived from Vedic astrology. These mantras are the cosmic signature of the stars and the unique vibration of the universe at the moment of one's birth. It is aligned to the light from the star that heralded as one entered into the manifest physical realm. [6] It is a unique and special way to practice mantra meditation that helps to peel back the years of conditioning and reveal a more authentic version of ourselves. These mantras are gifted by a teacher through a ceremony (look in the back of this book for a QR code that will lead you to receive your own Nakshatra Birthstar Mantra). There is a defined astrological meaning to the mantra. Still, meditators who use this style of mantra often practice disconnecting from the meaning and tapping into the vibration of the mantra instead. Some purposefully do not know the meaning of it as it can hinder the practice, while others find tremendous value in connecting with the meaning. The human mind likes to wrap meaning, thoughts, and results around words and practices. Disconnecting from the labels of our minds can be very powerful. In Sanskrit, the sound of any one mantra is more important than the meaning. It is said that a whispered mantra is 100 times more powerful than a spoken mantra, and a silent mantra is 1000 times more powerful than a whispered mantra.

Today, mantras have found their way from these ancient traditions into our modern world. Mantras come in many more forms and are mostly written in ancient or indigenous languages. However, mantras can also be practiced in the native tongue, and some affirmations are easily transferable to an English mantra practice. Thus, we can benefit from the ancient wisdom of mantras even today. They integrate well with holistic practices, as they consider all aspects of an individual, including the body, mind, and spirit. Throughout the book, you will be guided through simple affirmations and mantras, receive answers to all your questions, and feel better prepared to apply affirmations and mantras.

As we continue to learn more about affirmations and mantras, consider what areas of your life could be impacted by a positive practice. How could this help you co-create your life? How could personal fulfillment transpire using affirmations and mantras? Take a moment to write down some areas of your life that you would like to transform. Areas to consider can be: Health, wealth, purpose, mindset, emotions, passion, relationships, spirituality, and contribution.

Areas of Desired Transformation

_____

_____

_____

_____

_____

_____

_____

_____

_____

_____

_____

_____

THE SCIENCE BEHIND AFFIRMATIONS AND THEIR IMPACT ON THE MENTAL AND PHYSICAL BODY

For many of us, there are patterns and ways of being that we can't seem to change. Despite many attempts and the use of various modalities, we find ourselves in the same loops of negative thoughts, emotions, and behaviors. Affirmations can interrupt these automatic cycles of undesired patterns by reprogramming your subconscious mind and creating changes in the brain. The reason why change seems so difficult is that, over time, our subconscious mind becomes hardwired to think the same thoughts. It all starts in childhood, especially until the age of 7; our subconscious mind is very open and susceptible to the programs of our environment. Neural networks are formed that align with our habitual thoughts and behaviors. These are based on programs learned from parents, caregivers, and the general environment. For example, if you have heard repeatedly in your childhood that you are not good enough or you can't achieve your goals, this is rooted deeply in your subconscious mind and might affect your life today. Additionally, our subconscious mind, which relates to our beliefs, skills, self-image, memories, and more, is responsible for 90% of our behavior. Our conscious mind, which controls rational thinking such as the decision to change, only accounts for about 10%. [7] Can you see the reason why so many people are stuck in the same negative cycles? The conscious decision to change ourselves can't overcome our powerful subconscious mind unless we do the work to create change at that level.

This is exactly where the power of affirmations comes in. Whether you are aware of it or not, you are constantly talking with yourself via your thoughts. Your self-talk, which acts as affirmations, is either positive or negative, and it can help you create the life you desire or keep you stuck. The thoughts you think lead to actions, and with that, to a certain outcome or way of being in the world.

On the level of the brain, saying an affirmation activates the reticular activating system (RAS), known as the filter of our brain. With countless amounts of information and stimuli being directed toward us at every moment, the RAS decides which information is important and processes it further. [8] By repeating positive affirmations, we signal our brain that these words are important to us, and they sink deeper into our conscious and subconscious minds. Thus, our affirmations become part of our subconscious belief system, and we take aligned action on the conscious level.

Our subconscious mind learns through repetition; that's why repeating the affirmations many times is essential. Affirmations are not magic; they only work when we make them work.

Even studies show that self-affirmations work effectively. Research has indicated that affirmations can decrease stress, increase well-being, improve academic performance, and make people more open to behavior change. Results from one study showed that people who practiced affirmations focused on their future outcomes had increased activity in brain areas related to self-processing, which reflected in positive action in their physical lives. [9] Practicing affirmation helps us to see more possibilities in our dreams and goals and to make them a reality by taking action toward them. Self-affirmations can help us to break through self-sabotage and take aligned action because they replace negative thought patterns that are deeply ingrained in our subconscious mind with healthier ways of thinking. This positively influences our entire system, mind, and body. [10] On the level of the mind, scientists discovered that affirmations help us to realign with our core values and our natural states of self-worth. [11] Interestingly, this is closely related to the ancient *Nakshatra Birthstar Mantra* meditation, in which a mantra aligns an individual with their unique vibration at birth. When we are born, we are in a pure state of being in which love, worthiness, and alignment with the universe are natural. It is only when we grow up and are programmed that we start believing in negative patterns such as unworthiness. Affirmations help us restore our natural, vibrant selves.

Mantra Meditation (MM) has also been shown to be effective in helping with one of the biggest complaints in our modern society: Chronic stress, which is directly connected to six leading causes of death. Humans worldwide used to die of infections, and although modern medicine and lifestyle have greatly helped us in this arena, now our modern life has significantly increased stress, which leads to heart disease, hypertension, diabetes, depression, anxiety disorder, and more. [12] And, while research is still being conducted to see if stress causes cancer, it indeed inhibits the body from taking proper action on inhibiting or ridding the body of diseased cells. [13]

Scientific studies show that MM allows the body and mind to enter a space of profound rest. Heart rate and breathing can decrease, and there is a lower state of anxiety. [14] This deep rest experienced in MM prepares us with the tools needed to cope with stress as it arises during the day. It is widely known that people who have a consistent meditation practice cope with stress as more of a challenge rather than a problem. Thus, MM can protect us from the more detrimental effects that stress can have on our physical and emotional well-being.

Mantra meditation has also been found to sharply reduce anxiety and high blood pressure as it has a calming effect on the mind. [15] When we bring ourselves to the present moment with affirmations and mantras and continue to repeat them silently, we are no longer ruminating on the past or worrying about the future. We are concentrating on our words. This, again, acts as a pattern interrupt to a conditioned stress response that we have learned and picked up some time between birth and now. With what we know about stress and how it is a leading cause of death-related illnesses, the more we practice meditation, the more we reduce our stress, and the healthier we become - at the level of mind, body, and soul. Even science confirms that mantra meditation is one of the most effective meditation techniques in today's world. [16]

THE EFFECTIVENESS OF AFFIRMATIONS

Jane had always struggled with self-doubt and insecurity despite her professional achievements. She often found herself comparing her progress to others and feeling inadequate, which hindered her ability to pursue her career goals with confidence. She often felt imposter syndrome even though she had been rewarded for a job well done. Jane was able to trace this pattern back to her childhood, in which she was repeatedly told by caregivers that her results at school were not enough, that she should achieve higher grades like her siblings did, and that otherwise, she couldn't achieve success. Although Jane was very aware of this pattern, she was unsure how to transform it after trying to create change for many years. When learning about the power of affirmations, she rewrote these negative beliefs into more positive ones. For example, the belief "Your results are not good enough. You can't achieve success" was rewritten into "I am enough and worthy just as I am. I am successful at whatever I do." She repeated this affirmation in the morning and evening and at other times throughout the day. In the beginning, there was a lot of resistance for Jane, as this affirmation didn't feel true to her. But she persisted, and after a few weeks, she started to feel the truth of this new affirmation in her heart. First, her inner reality and then her outer reality started to transform. By shifting her mindset and embracing a more positive outlook through the power of self-affirmation, she was able to overcome her self-doubt, achieve greater success in her career, and experience a newfound sense of confidence and fulfillment in all areas of her life.

In the next chapter, you will learn how to create your own personal affirmations to transform any area of your life.

CHAPTER TWO
CRAFTING POWERFUL AFFIRMATIONS

> "When you do things from your soul, you feel a river of joy within you."
> — *Rumi*

What if you could create your own affirmations? You have searched and scrolled through affirmations to support your unique desires, but there does not seem to be one that resonates. This is not to say they are not good affirmations, but they are not for you. We all have our unique patterns we wish to change, our own desires, goals, and dreams. The most powerful affirmations are the ones that feel aligned for us. Where to even begin?

PRINCIPLES OF CRAFTING EFFECTIVE AFFIRMATIONS

Some general principles unlock the power of self-affirmation. [1] Working with affirmations isn't just about repeating any statement robotically - there are certain nuances that make an affirmation powerful and effective.

Get specific: The more general you are, the less impactful an affirmation can be. What is the end result? Make the affirmation specific to your situation. Do not focus on how to get there but on the specific end result. For example, instead of "I do what I like and increase my income," say, "I am creating my own soul-aligned business and have an extra income of $500 a month."

Use Positive Words: Refrain from using words like "don't" or "won't". The universe does not understand contractions like this. If you were to say, "I don't want to gain more weight," you would basically be saying, "Hey universe, add some more weight, please!" Instead, say something like, "I am healthy and fit and am at my ideal size." See the difference?

Use present tense: Instead of, "I will be fit and healthy," say, "I *am* fit and healthy." Say it and feel it as if it's already done. Your subconscious mind doesn't know the difference between imagination and reality. If you affirm something in the present tense, your subconscious will assume it's true and help you to create it.

Make your affirmation resonate: If it does not feel right, craft it until it does. The affirmation should feel empowering, uplifting, and true to you. If there is any resistance when you start saying the affirmation, that's fine. You are changing a deeply ingrained pattern. Look for a deeper truth in your heart as to whether the affirmation feels right.

Be succinct: Keep it short and sweet. When we over-explain, we get into the minutiae, which could be called getting stuck in the mud. Again, don't try to figure out "the how"; just assume it is done. Mike Dooley, author of Infinite Possibilities and more, famously calls the details of "hows" the "curse-ed hows." Don't do it. The affirmation will become complicated, and you will become frustrated.

TRY IT: Now that you understand the principles of successful affirmations, you can create your own affirmations to change your life step by step.

1. Choose one area of your life that you would like to change. It could be one of the areas you chose in the previous chapter.

    For example: Wealth

2. Create awareness. What is your current self-talk in this area of your life? What are you saying to yourself daily?

    For example: I can observe that I constantly say that I don't have enough money to do what I really want to do. I keep complaining about my day job and that I want to start a meaningful business, but I keep talking myself out of starting it. I tell myself that I can't do it, that I'm not good enough. I can see that I don't feel worthy of being financially wealthy.

3. What are your results? Can you see a connection between your thoughts and the outcomes?

    For example: I live paycheck to paycheck and have enough money to get by, but I want more from life than just working a job I don't enjoy. When I reflect on this, I know I am here for something more meaningful.

4. Write down your current thoughts or negative beliefs.

    For example: I don't feel worthy of being wealthy. I believe I am not good enough and can't start my own business.

5. Transform these beliefs into positive affirmations that feel true to you. These statements should reflect who you truly are at the core of your being.

    For example: I am enough just as I am. I am worthy of financial abundance. I am successful and have a blossoming online business doing what I love, and create an extra income of $1000 a month.

6. Bonus: Write down how you feel when your affirmation comes true, and truly FEEL it now.

    For example: It feels liberating and purposeful to have my own business and to live in financial abundance. It is wonderful!

Using this process and the previous areas of life that you would like to transform. Take a few moments to craft a personal affirmation in each area of transformation.

_____

_____

_____

_____

_____

_____

_____

_____

_____

_____

_____

_____

_____

_____

_____

_____

_____

_____

_____

When you have your affirmations ready, it's time to start practicing. Set a reminder on your phone, something gentle and easy, and start practicing your affirmations three to five minutes a day. My husband likes to write post-it notes with his affirmations on them and places them in the bathroom mirror, on his desk, and where he often sees them. However, this can become something the brain looks over, so even if you place them on post-it notes to read, it is important to set a time to practice them daily. Some ideas:

- Practice affirmations in the morning right when you get up and in the evening just before sleep. These are the times of the day when the subconscious mind is most susceptible to being reprogrammed.
- You can also practice during any activity in your day-to-day life. Repeat your affirmations while showering, making your breakfast, driving to work, going for a walk, and exercising.
- When there is space in your schedule, sit down, take some deep breaths, and get a clear vision of your affirmation in your mind's eye. See what the ideal outcome is. Once you get a clear vision in your head, start repeating your affirmation over and over to yourself. You can do this in an audible voice, a whisper, or in silence. Do what is easiest for you and feels the best. Raise your words, not your voice. As Rumi said: *"It is rain that grows flowers, not thunder."*

Don't be discouraged if, in the beginning, you find it difficult to feel the truth of your affirmations. Resistance is there because the affirmation takes you "out of your comfort zone"; it is different from what your subconscious mind is used to affirm. And our subconscious mind loves what is familiar and keeps us safe in our comfort zone. However, as you might have experienced yourself, if we want to unfold our fullest potential and become the truest version of ourselves, we have to step out of this comfort zone. If you experience resistance, embrace it and see it as a sign that you are heading in the right direction - the direction of your truth. Keep going with repeating your affirmations, as eventually, you will be able to feel the truth of what you affirm with your entire being. This is usually the point when the transformation happens; we become our affirmation. Our inner state is changed, and it reflects in our outer world. *"As within, so without."*

ALIGNING AFFIRMATIONS WITH THE SEVEN MAIN CHAKRAS

You can go further in creating affirmations and align them with the seven main chakra systems. Chakra is a Sanskrit word for "circle" or "wheel". They are energy centers found within us all and assist in balancing both mental and physical health through energy. [2] These energy centers are situated along the spine and correlate with different organs, energies, and qualities. Each Chakra can be balanced or blocked. When a chakra is balanced, this means life force energy, or *prana*, is flowing freely, and the qualities associated with the chakra can be expressed. When a chakra is blocked, the energy is stagnant and can't flow through the body.

Depending on your current inner work, you can use affirmations to align with a different chakra statement. [3]

The **Root Chakra**, or *Muladhara Chakra*, is located at the perineum and is associated with the color red. This is a primal chakra and, when balanced, brings about groundedness, energy, physical fitness, safety, security, calm, centeredness, and fearlessness. I am statements such as, "I am healthy and fit" or "I am safe, sound, and secure in every way," are grounding root chakra affirmations. If you are someone who has a hard time staying grounded and "spaces out" often or people tell you things like, "Your head is always in the clouds," you may benefit from grounding affirmations such as these.

The **Sacral Chakra**, or *Svadhistana Chakra*, is located in the lower abdomen close to the sexual organs and is associated with the color orange. It's related to our sexual energy, emotions, creativity, and fluidity. This chakra helps us to regulate our emotions and desires and to express our creativity. I feel statements such as "I feel creative, aligned with my infinite potential" or "I feel deeply connected and in tune with my emotions and desires" are sacral chakra affirmations. If you feel blocked in expressing your creativity, find it difficult to regulate your emotions, or if you feel disconnected from your sexual energy, you might want to work with sacral chakra affirmations.

The **Solar Plexus Chakra**, or *Manipura Chakra*, is situated in the navel center and relates to the color yellow. It's connected to our power, inner strength, and determination. It also relates to our self-confidence and our ability to take action. I do statements such as "I do express my power, confidence and I can handle anything" or "I do embrace my power and assert myself confidently in the world" are examples of solar plexus chakra affirmations. If you experience anger issues, digestive problems, depression, or a lack of self-esteem, it can be helpful to work with this chakra.

The **Heart Chakra**, or *Anahata Chakra*, is situated in the heart center and is associated with the color green. It's connected to unconditional love, peace, and trust. It is said to be the home of our higher, infinite self, and it is connected to the relationship we have with ourselves and others. I love statements such as "I love myself and others" or "I love to create peace in the world", which are heart chakra affirmations. If you feel that the flow of love in your life is blocked, if you experience anxiety, jealousy, or fear, this can be a sign to open your heart chakra.

The **Throat Chakra**, or *Vishudda Chakra*, is located in the throat area and is associated with the color blue. Its qualities are spiritual aspiration, purity, healthy self-expression, and authenticity. It helps us to share our true voice with the world. I speak statements such as "I speak my truth" or "I speak only what is an authentic expression of myself" are throat chakra affirmations. If you feel an inability to express yourself or a sense of disconnection from your truth and authenticity, throat chakra affirmations can be beneficial.

The **Third Eye Chakra**, or *Ajna Chakra*, is in the middle of the forehead between the eyebrows. Its colors are indigo. The qualities of this chakra are intuition, vision, and self-knowledge. Statements such as "I see a clear vision for my life" or "I see myself as I really am" are third-eye chakra affirmations. If you experience confusion, headaches, or blurry vision, you may benefit from third-eye chakra affirmations.

The **Crown Chakra**, or *Sahasrara Chakra*, is situated on the crown of the head. Its associated color is ultra-violet (all colors). Sahasrara Chakra is connected with oneness, inner peace, self-mastery, and divine energies. I know statements such as "I know the wisdom of divine consciousness" or "I know peace within myself" are examples of crown chakra affirmations. If you feel disconnected from life, frustrated, or experiencing melancholy, you might want to work with crown chakra affirmations.

Root Chakra: I Am

Sacral Chakra: I Feel

Solar Plexus Chakra: I Do

Heart Center Chakra: I Love

Throat Chakra: I Speak

Third Eye Chakra: I See

Crown Chakra: I Know

TRY IT: Take some time to reflect on the different areas of your life, and try to understand which chakras might be out of balance. For example, if you don't feel satisfied in the area of wealth, explore the deeper causes. Are you not feeling safe to receive money? Then, create a root chakra affirmation, such as " I am safe to receive financial abundance." Are you feeling unable to take action to increase your finances? Come up with a solar plexus chakra affirmation, such as: "I do act on my inspiration and dreams and can attract more money with joy." If you feel blocked in the area of relationships, you may want to work with a heart chakra affirmation, like "I love myself and others. I give and receive love freely." "Make sure that any chakra affirmation relates to your unique situation and feels good and true. You can follow the basic steps mentioned earlier in this chapter to create your chakra affirmations.

I Am

_____

_____

_____

I Feel

_____

_____

_____

_____

I Do

_____

_____

_____

_____

I Love

_____

_____

_____

_____

I Speak

_____

_____

_____

_____

I See

_____

_____

_____

_____

I Know

_____

_____

_____

_____

A SUCCESSFUL INDIVIDUAL USING CUSTOMIZED AFFIRMATIONS

Sarah had always struggled with self-doubt and insecurity. No matter how hard she tried, she couldn't shake off the negative thoughts that seemed to cloud her mind. She felt like she couldn't express her authentic self and found herself stuck in people-pleasing and playing small in all areas of her life. Feeling stuck and unhappy with her life, she decided that enough was enough. She was determined to make a change and take control of her thoughts. She did some research and started crafting her own affirmations to help build her confidence and self-esteem. She came up with affirmations such as "I am enough, just as I am. I embrace my flaws and celebrate my strengths." or "I fully express my power and live as my most authentic self." She also added some specific throat chakra and solar plexus affirmations, such as "I speak my truth with confidence and joy" and "I do what I love and enjoy, not what others want me to do." In the beginning, Sarah felt uncomfortable saying these affirmations, as they were so different from her usual self-talk. But she shared that deep inside, she felt a spark light up as she internalized these affirmations. Deep in her heart, she felt these words express who she really is at her core. After her first month of self-affirming, Sarah noticed remarkable changes in her life. She felt much more confident in herself; she was able to set boundaries and say "no," and she started to feel so much more comfortable being herself. After two months, she gained so much momentum that she started to train as a transformational coach, as she desired to help other women break out of the cycle of smallness, insecurity, and people-pleasing. Today, many months later, she has a successful coaching business and feels happy and fulfilled with her life.

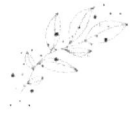

CHAPTER THREE
THE ART OF MANTRAS

"The lamps are different but the light is the same."
— *Rumi*

Mantras and Mantra Meditation are genuinely some of my favorite things in life. The power of a mantra is profound as we connect to the vibration and let go of the meaning. Mantras are a sacred and individual practice that can calm the storm within and help us to disconnect from the chaos of life and access the stillness and silence that rests within. Mantras are often partnered with mala beads or mudras. Let's explore more.

EXPLORING THE ORIGINS AND MEANINGS OF MANTRAS

In today's world, you might hear modern coaches and pop culture say, "Simply find your mantra and use it." In truth, mantras are not as simple as that. They are much more sacred and have to be understood in depth to unfold their power. A mantra can be a single word or, more often, a sound or group of words. The word mantra originates from the Sanskrit expression "man," which means "to think."[1] A mantra can thus be understood as an instrument of thought.[2] However, mantras point to a different way of thinking than is commonly known in the Western world. Usually, our thinking is very scattered; it is automatic, and we tend to think thoughts that don't serve us. With mantras, our entire attention is focused on one single thought: the mantra. This means we disconnect from the usual chaos of our thoughts and become completely immersed in the mantra. We don't even use thoughts to understand the meaning of a mantra; rather, we connect to the sound of a mantra and let go of any attempts to understand the meaning. This can lead to profound states of transcendence, to *gnosis* or divine inner knowing beyond ordinary thoughts, and helps us to think more clearly in daily life.

The concept of mantras originated in the Vedic period (1000 B.C.E. - 500 B.C.E.), during which people started chanting mantras during their meditation practice. [3] Mantras evolved from three Vedic texts: *Rig Veda, Samur Veda*, and *Yajur Veda*. Today, people still use mantras from these ancient texts. Mantras can come in many languages; however, Sanskrit mantras tend to be more well-known internationally. Over the years, the practice of mantras grew from a small group of practitioners to now being a regular practice for millions of people worldwide. This shows how relevant and beneficial mantras are in today's modern world. The chanting of a mantra out loud, as a whisper, or silently to yourself can help our physical, psychological, emotional, and spiritual well-being. They can calm and soothe the mind, be used to raise our vibration, balance the chakras, help us improve concentration, keep us in the present moment, reduce stress, and even help us fall asleep at night.

Mantras can be woven into your daily practice in many ways, depending on your preferences. As always, finding a way that truly resonates with you is important.

In Japa meditation, mala beads are used with a mantra. I received my first mala in 2018 and loved using it. Now, I can't stop collecting malas. They are a sacred and spiritual tool to use during meditation. Mala beads are a sacred tool that becomes infused with every mantra uttered aloud, in a whisper, or silently over and over to yourself. I know some people who will keep those malas with them for when they experience stress during the day. As they do, they take a few moments to step away, use a mantra, and bring themselves into the present moment. A mala consists of 108 beads, as 108 is seen as a sacred number in Hinduism.[4] The number 108 represents universal consciousness as the essence of everything, symbolized as one (1), nothing

(0), and everything (8 or infinity).[5] Therefore, the 108 Mala beads remind us that we are all Divine consciousness expressed as form. The significance of the number 108 reaches outside of Hinduism - there are even 108 stitches on a baseball, and a few times a year, we are 108 suns away from the sun, and on its respective days, we are 108 moons away from the moon itself.[6]

Japa meditation is a great way to time yourself without technology and aid your meditation with another point of focus and gentle concentration. To use a mala, you can let it rest over the third finger of the right hand and bring the beads toward you, counting them one by one, using the thumb. With each bead you touch, you repeat the mantra one time. When you touch the guru bead, you stop in devotion to your inner or outer guru (a.k.a. spiritual teacher) and then start counting the beads in the other direction.[7] You can choose a specific mantra for your mala beads practice based on your intention. As you repeat the mantra with each bead, there will be a harmonious rhythm that allows you to enter a state of meditation.[8] It is important to choose a mantra that deeply resonates with you. The right mantra for you should feel aligned; its repetition feels effortless and harmonious, the mantra captures your attention, you feel a sense of wonderment, and it helps you to go deeper within by calming your mind. Besides choosing your mantra, you can also decide to follow one of three types of Japa Meditation: In *Maanas Meditation*, you repeat the mantra silently in your mind; in *Vachak Meditation*, you say or chant the mantra in a low voice; and during *Kirtan Meditation*, you chant the mantra out loud.[9]

Another form of mantra meditation is using OM as your mantra. OM is both a sound or mantra and a visual symbol. In Hinduism, the sound of OM is a primordial sound or vibration, and from this first vibration, all sounds originate.[10] OM consists of three sounds: A, U, and M – AUM, which represent the three vibrations that are inherent in the creation of the universe.[11] "A" is seen as the beginning of the universe, the starting point of creation. "U" represents the energy that preserves and carries creation forward in the physical world. "M" symbolizes the dissolution of the manifest world back into spirit.[12] Traditionally, OM is chanted three times as a reminder of the three meanings of AUM, and to harmonize the three parts of our being—the mind, body, and spirit.[13] Often, meditators will use OM as their mantra, such as Om Moksha Ritam. OM is considered the hymn of the universe heralding our Oneness, and it has even been studied to find that it is a brain stabilizer that invokes calm, especially when stress is present. This has been confirmed by Indian scientists. [14]

OM, as a visual symbol, represents five states of consciousness. The lower left curve symbolizes the waking state of being. The top left curve represents the unconscious state. The lower right curve is the dream state—the state between the waking and the unconscious. The semicircle at the top is the Maya state, which means the veil of illusion. The dot at the top symbolizes the absolute or transcendental state, the pure bliss of just being.[15]

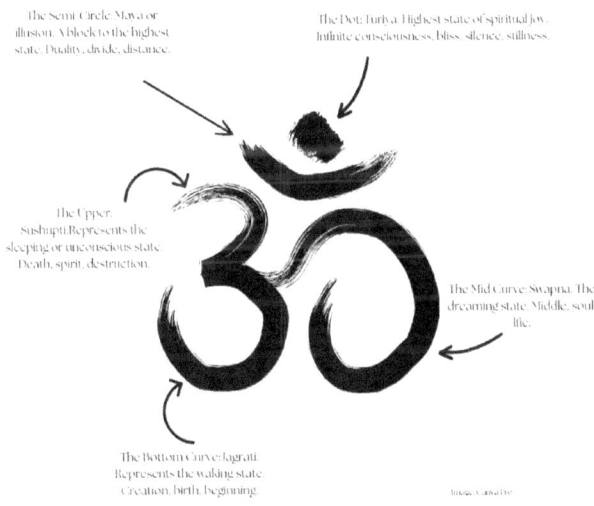

INCORPORATING MANTRAS INTO DAILY PRACTICE FOR SPIRITUAL AND EMOTIONAL GROWTH

In essence, there are three ways to incorporate mantras into your daily practice.

The first way is to use mantras on an "as-needed" basis. When the mind chatter gets too loud, you are having a stressful day, or you experience a lot of anxiety, you can practice repeating a mantra silently or out loud. It can calm the mind, take you back into the present moment, and into feelings of peace and relaxation.[16]

The second way is to incorporate mantras into your daily meditation routine. You can chant a mantra at the beginning or end or have a section of your meditation practice dedicated to chanting mantras. For example, you could begin each meditation by chanting OM three times and end a session by chanting your favorite mantra.

The third way is a dedicated 40-day mantra practice. You choose one mantra and repeat it every day 108 times with your mala beads for 40 continuous days.[17] This is a great way to fuel your inner fire and aspiration for your practice and create a new habit. It is recommended for more advanced practitioners, who already have a daily mantra practice.

No matter what way you choose - the essence of mantras and affirmations is to transform your daily life. If you are not sure how they can support you and what their function is, then this section is for you. Most people experience a gap in their lives - between where they currently are, their circumstances, and their ideal life. For people who are on a spiritual path, their ideal life is usually based on their hearts' purpose, their mission in life, and the expression of their highest self. For example, you might find yourself habitually doubting yourself and playing small, whereas, in your heart, you know that you came here to express authentically and share your gifts. Or, you might find yourself in a job that just pays the bills but doesn't feel fulfilling, and you know you are here to create a purposeful business. Or, you keep finding yourself attracting the same unavailable partners, whereas you desire a committed, loving relationship. It doesn't matter what gap you experience; mantras and affirmations help you to bridge the gap from where you are to where you are longing to be. The reason why so many people wish to transform their lives but feel stuck is because their destructive thoughts and behaviors have become so habitual that they are challenging to change. To create lasting transformation, we have to change the paradigm of our life; we have to change the concept we have of ourselves. If our idea of ourselves is based on the conditioning of the subconscious mind we received as a child, then we must change this conditioning at the level of the subconscious mind.

By repeating affirmations and chanting mantras often, daily, the chanter creates new neural pathways in your brain, and change the content of your subconscious mind and, thus, your self-concept. You start speaking differently to yourself and others; you feel differently and make new choices. For example, if you are longing to attract a healthy, romantic relationship, but your automatic inner self-talk consists of sentences like "I'm not lovable," "Men/women don't like me as I am.", "Men/women always hurt me," you are not in the state of being able to attract an emotionally available partner into your life. By becoming aware of these words, changing them, and creating new affirmations such as "I am loveable. Men/women love getting to know my authentic self. I am safe to love and be loved," you transform yourself in resonance with a healthy, loving relationship.

The transformation you can experience in any aspect of your daily life might feel almost magical; however, it is even backed up by science. Mantras are known to induce a state of deeper awareness, helping us to observe our thoughts without judgments, regulate our emotions, and even counteract stress. One study found that mantra meditation reduces stress levels, improves psychological resilience, and helps individuals deal with challenging situations [18] Another study showed that repeating mantras induces deep states of relaxation and activates the parasympathetic nervous system, which calms the body and reduces the levels of stress hormones in the body. [19] This means that mantra meditation can help with one of the most significant threats in our modern life: chronic, daily stress. Another study showed that mantra meditation can help people cultivate non-judgment towards their thoughts and emotions and deepen self-awareness. [20]

Thus, repeating mantras opens us up to a relaxed state of being from which we can observe our habitual thoughts and emotions and change them. Additionally, mantras can help us with specific problems we might encounter in daily life. For example, you might want to forgive someone or find it challenging, or you feel strong emotional or physical pain and would like to release it. Or, you would like to feel more connected to your higher self. There is a mantra for whatever circumstance you might find yourself in. Are you feeling curious about finding a mantra that resonates with you or helps you deal with a specific circumstance in your life?

At the end of this book, you will find many different mantra ideas to choose from. Here are some examples so you can get started with your practice right away, depending on your current state of being and intentions.

For spiritual growth

- *Om So Hum* ="I am That". To connect with the universe, regulate your breathing and soothe your mind
- *Om Namah Shivaya* = "I bow to the inner Self/Pure Consciousness/Shiva". A famous Hindu mantra evoking pure consciousness.

For forgiveness and compassion:

- *Om Mani Padme Hum* = "On the path of life, with intention and wisdom, we can achieve the pure body, speech, and mind of a Buddha." It is used for enhancing feelings of compassion and love and is a very common mantra in Buddhism.
- *Lokah Samastah Sukhino Bhavantu* = "May all beings everywhere be happy and free, and may the thoughts, words, and actions of my own life contribute in some way to that happiness and to that freedom for all." It's a mantra to dissolve the ego self and radiate positive energy to all beings

To heal pain and suffering

- *Tayata Om Bekandze Bekandze* = "May the many sentient beings who are sick, be freed from sickness soon. And may all the sicknesses of beings never arise again." It's known as the Medicine Buddha mantra and heals pain and suffering.

FINDING SOLACE THROUGH MANTRA MEDITATION

When I first started meditating, mantras were far, far away. If you read my first book, then you know that body scans were my introduction to the world of meditation. Mantras did not come until later when a lot of my pain and trauma was healing. At first, I found them awkward, and truthfully, I did not like saying them. When doing my morning ritual and listening to guided meditations by my teacher, davidji, chanting "OM" out loud at the end of the meditation made me feel uncomfortable even though I was just by myself. My dog would look at me curiously, then quickly lay back down. But as I kept coming back and meditating day after day, gradually, the mantras, the chanting, and the OM's helped me to transform. Mantras became part of my daily practice. But it did not stop there; mantras became my way of staying present when the chatter would not stop. You know, the chatter of the mind, the persistent, loud-mouthed, unmatched wittiness of letting the train of thought barrel down the tracks well over the posted speed. I can honestly say that today, this mind chatter and chaos is very rarely my state of consciousness. It still happens, and I am still growing in my practice (do we ever stop?), but that kind of chatter does not present itself often. In fact, runaway chatter during the day is virtually non-existent. Chatter mostly happens during the magic hour of 2:00 a.m., even though it is not anywhere close to what it used to be. Now, I use different mantras for different times of the day. I also use my Nakshatra Birthstar Mantra consistently. When the night-time "what-ifs" crawl in my ear, and I find myself lying in bed with my eyes wide open, my current mantra of choice is the ancient Hawaiian mantra, *Ho'opono opono*, which means: I'm sorry. Please forgive me. Thank you. I love you.[21] It's the most beautiful mantra for the reconciliation of loved ones and owning our part to play in every situation, no matter if we feel justified in our actions. I would rather feel peace and love rather than feel "I'm right and you're wrong." Being right is not what it's cracked up to be. My point in all this is that I have used mantras for anything we could face in this modern world, from reducing my stress at the airport, getting over "that thing" that just upset me while walking around the grocery store, to lifting my mood when I need an attitude adjustment. It is a deeply personal and sacred practice that has become interwoven in every aspect of my life, and I'm far better because of it.

CHAPTER FOUR

USING AFFIRMATIONS FOR SELF-LOVE, PROSPERITY AND SUCCESS

> "Yesterday I was clever so I wanted to change the world, today I am wise so I am changing myself."
> — *Rumi*

> "Your task is not to seek for love, but merely to seek and find all the barriers within yourself that you have built against it."
> — *Rumi*

THE TRUE MEANING OF SELF-LOVE AND PROSPERITY

Ultimately, we all long to truly love ourselves. To be so filled with love that we can share it with others and bring more love into the world. Commonly, self-love is seen as a state of appreciating oneself, which is expressed in actions that enhance our physical, psychological, and spiritual growth.[1] Self-love means we prioritize our own well-being, needs, and boundaries rather than sacrificing our truth to please others.[2] All success in life is the natural result of having a loving relationship with ourselves. In fact, nothing in this world can be better than the relationship we have with ourselves. Until we find and heal the barriers within ourselves that we have built against love, we will search the world for the love that can only be found within. We look for things, people, and situations to make us feel happy, loved, and accepted finally. But this is our responsibility. And the moment we take responsibility for our relationship with ourselves and feel determined to change it, life truly begins. What is essential for developing self-love is a deeper connection with our hearts. According to a study done in 1991, the heart is actually our little brain and has 40,000 neurons that think and learn, just like those neurons of the brain. The heart actually sends more information to the brain than the brain sends to the heart... like 80%.[3] When there is coherence, a harmonious connection between the heart and the brain, we can easily access what is true for us in any given situation. The heart is like an organ of knowledge; it contains a deeper knowing, an intuition about what decisions to make and how to move forward with our lives. Rather than staying at the level of the mind and rationally weighing all the different options, our heart naturally knows what is true for us.[4]

To connect with our heart, it is essential to become still. To stop the noise and chatter in our minds and to bring all of our attention to our hearts. You can do this by placing one hand on your heart or even taking a few deep breaths into your heart. Then, let your heart expand and allow warmth, softness, and love to arise. Once you feel connected with your heart, you can ask any question and allow for an answer to emerge. Often, it's a gentle whisper, a feeling, or a resonance. Sometimes, our heart feels open to an option; sometimes, it feels contracted. After a while, you will know how your heart communicates with you.

With this, it is crucial to understand what self-love truly means to you - in your heart. For some people, it can mean developing a more intimate relationship with themselves and to romanticize their lives. For others, it means being nice to themselves, engaging in a self-care routine, setting healthy boundaries, forgiving themselves, taking better care of their bodies, or resting more. For some, it means making changes to their lives - doing more things they love, starting a new creative endeavor, finally starting therapy, or getting a job where they feel appreciated.

Exercise: What does self-love truly mean to you?

You will now be guided to connect more deeply with your meaning for self-love, as it is at this very moment. There is no right or wrong or a specific way you should feel about it. All that matters is that it's an authentic expression of you. We will also practice connecting you with your heart. Find a comfortable space to sit in a comfortable position. Place one hand on your heart and connect with the love within you. For a few moments, rest in this connection with your heart. Then, evoke the question: "What does my heart truly long for in regards to self-love?" Let the answer arise from your heart, your intuition, a deeper part of your being. Take note of whatever comes up. Also, stay alert and receptive during your day, as the answer might surface later. If an answer does not arise within a day or two, keep asking. The more you ask, the better we get at receiving the answer.

Besides self-love, it seems like everyone in today's world is speaking about wealth. These days, social media is filled with tutorials on how to grow passive income, double our earnings, or even become a millionaire. Money is the currency on this planet and, as such, deserves our attention. Most people want to have more money in their lives but feel unable to achieve it. Those on a spiritual path often want to live their true purpose but find themselves unable to because they are working a stressful job to provide for their needs. If you find financial limitations in your life, again, this is likely rooted in the subconscious mind. If you learned in childhood that you don't deserve money, that money is evil or the root of all problems, or if you heard the common phrase "You have to work hard for money" over and over again, chances are that these beliefs are reflected in your relationship with money today. The truth is that our natural state of being is abundance. We live in a world of infinite possibilities and abundance. It all starts by harnessing inner abundance and becoming an abundant person. Naturally, this will reflect in abundance in the outer world. In his book "The Power of Now," Eckhart Tolle introduces the parable of the beggar and the box of gold. He tells the story of a man who sat on the side of the road for over 30 years, begging people for money. One day, a stranger asked the man: "What is inside the box you are sitting on? Have you ever looked inside?" The beggar replied that there was no point in looking inside as there was nothing in the box. After the stranger insists, the beggar opens the box and finds, with astonishment, that it is full of gold.[5] This parable implies that the box of gold is within us, not in the outer world. Once we rest in the prosperity of our being, we will live in a prosperous world.

Still, it is important to decide what abundance and prosperity truly mean to you. It's different for everyone. Some people say we should be as prosperous as we can, and some people say we should be content with as little as possible. For a single mom, abundance could mean going to the grocery store and not worrying about staying within budget. For a businessman, abundance could mean scaling to millions of dollars to buy that 2nd home with a boat and other toys in the garage. For another person, it could mean living a life in alignment with their soul and creating money from sharing their gifts rather than working a job they don't enjoy. Abundance, for me, is freedom of time, freedom of location, and freedom of finances.

The important question is: What does abundance truly mean for you?

Exercise: What does abundance truly mean to your heart?

Once you feel ready to journey deeper into your meaning of abundance, find a comfortable and calm space to practice this exercise. Again, place one hand on your heart and connect with the depth of your being. For a few moments, rest in this connection with your heart. Then, evoke the question: "What does my heart truly long for regarding abundance?" Let the answers bubble up gently and easily. It's okay if they do not come right away; they may come later in the day. Write down whatever comes up for you.

_____

_____

_____

_____

_____

_____

_____

_____

HARNESSING AFFIRMATIONS FOR SELF-LOVE AND PROSPERITY

Why does it seem so hard for most people to love themselves, and how do we deepen into authentic self-love? Why do people say they want more money but can't seem to get out of financial limitations? As you might recall from Chapter One, we all were conditioned in childhood, and many of us have internalized programs such as not being worthy, being a failure, or not being wanted in our subconscious mind. Most adults still act from these same unconscious programs. Over time, these programs crystallize into strong patterns of thought, feeling, and behavior - they become our state of being, our personality. They become deeply ingrained in our subconscious mind, and neural networks in our brains are hardwired to keep us in this state of being unless we change these patterns. Thus, if you learned in childhood that you are not a good person, chances are you have difficulties loving yourself. If you learned that you don't deserve money, you likely get rid of your money every month rather than growing wealth. If you have learned that you are not good enough, you most likely can't seem to achieve the success you desire deep down.

The most important way these patterns limit our ability to love ourselves and to live the life of our dreams is through negative self-talk. Whether you are aware of it or not, you are constantly speaking with yourself through your thoughts. Just watch yourself on the way to work... Are you talking yourself down? What are you saying to yourself? Are you speaking negatively or positively to yourself? Self-talk is the automatic and repetitive use of cue words in a silent or vocalized dialog with oneself.[6] Talking to oneself is a habit everyone engages in; it is as natural as talking to a friend or engaging in our daily activities. Therefore, as we have so many thoughts and conversations with ourselves every day, rather than stopping this self-talk, what we want to do is become aware of it and control it. Most of us are completely unaware of our inner talking and of the fact that this self-talk creates our reality.

Self-talk is so powerful that it is commonly used for performance enhancement for professional athletes, in academic settings, and even in clinical environments to help regulate anxiety, depression, and other psychological issues.[7] Self-talk with positive content can help promote beneficial psychological states and regulate cognitions; it can increase our confidence and ability to take action towards our dreams and to achieve success in life. In contrast, self-talk with negative content is associated with decreased emotional well-being and self-criticism. Studies show that negative self-talk causes stress and anxiety, by activating the threat system in the body and that it leads to diminished self-confidence.[8] It's the chatter or the commonly uttered "Why in the hell did you do that, you idiot?" which is self-imposed. This has a strong negative mental and physical impact. In essence, every thought we have about ourselves acts as an affirmation. The good news is... You can change your inner self-talk and, with that, change your life and enhance your ability to create self-love, abundance, and success! Now that we know what self-love and prosperity mean to us on an intimate level and have also learned about the power of negative self-talk, let's get into rewiring our brains to have positive self-talk, step by step.

1. AWARENESS OF OLD PATTERNS

Observe what you say to yourself daily. Things like "That's too expensive, I cannot afford it" translate to I am not enough and reaffirm the lack in your life instead of abundance. Do you get mad at wealthy people? Do they upset you? If they do, that points to a strong limiting belief. Do you keep saying to yourself that you should be further ahead, that you are failing, or that you are stuck? This reflects a pattern of not loving and accepting yourself. It can be helpful to write down the stories you constantly tell yourself.

2. FORMING NEW AFFIRMATIONS

It is crucial to choose what you want to think. What thoughts and affirmations reflect the true you and the life you desire to create for yourself? For this step, use the lines below and if you need additional room, pull out a piece of paper. On the left side, write all the thoughts and patterns you think habitually, which you discovered in step one. For example, "I don't have enough money". On the right side, write the opposite of it, an affirmation that feels true and expansive for you. For example, "I always have enough money." or "There is always enough because I am enough". Listen to your heart and continue like this for all the patterns you became aware of.

(Seriously, stop and do this exercise)

Exercise: Habitual Negative Self-Talk

Opposite and Positive Affirmation

Negative Self Talk	*Positive Affirmation*

3. PATTERN INTERRUPT

Every time you hear criticism from yourself or others, change your stance with a pattern interruption. This means, in your daily life, you replace the patterns from step one, with the new patterns from step two. For example, if you become aware of a thought about lack, say "I am happy that I can circulate wealth and have financial freedom. I have financial freedom." When that little mean voice pops up and says you are not good enough, say "I am lovable and perfect as I am. I am loved and appreciated. I love and appreciate myself." The more your new pattern enforces a more positive narrative, the more your brain and thoughts will join that lane rather than the mean and negative one. If you find it difficult to interrupt your patterns, go back to step one, and deepen your awareness of your habitual thoughts. If any negative thought pattern is very strong, you can interrupt it by saying "Stop" or "Change" whenever it comes up, and then replacing it with your positive pattern. Be patient with yourself; results and changes come with time and repetition.

4. GRATITUDE

Have a gratitude practice and be thankful for everything you do have. Studies have shown that gratitude improves one's overall outlook on life as we focus on what's good and positive in our lives. It also helps us see that our lives would not be possible without the help of others.

5. DEVELOP A POSITIVE MINDSET

You can do all the affirmations out there, but if you find a problem for every solution, then you will continually see them. Affirmations are great, but action is required to look at yourself as a whole person. See how to shed the conditioning that sees the problem, rather than the action of solving it. [9] This also means surrounding yourself with abundance-minded people with similar optimistic, solution seekers. There is no time for people who have a problem for every solution. If you tend to be that way, practice seeing the possibilities rather than the limitations. Becoming more solution-minded is a priority. It keeps you from dwelling on the problem and looking in an expansive way to solve the issue. [10]

6. DEVELOP HEALTHY HABITS

Be sure to get enough sleep and follow a healthy routine. Having a routine for sleep, eating, affirmations, meditation, gratitude, time with loved ones, creativity, and hobbies can greatly impact keeping a healthy mindset and make it much easier to pattern interrupt negative talk to create new neural pathways. When we have a routine, we just do it without thinking about it. Meditation for me is a routine. I get up every morning, go pee, let my dogs pee, and feed them so they will relax and meditate. My teacher refers to this as R.P.M. Rise. Pee. Meditate. After this, I drink my greens and do some exercise. It's automatic as it is my routine that is established. It's my proverbial cup of coffee and starts my day out in a positive way.

REACHING A LEVEL OF ABUNDANCE AND PROSPERITY ON A NOT-SO-LARGE SCALE USING AFFIRMATIONS

One of my students, Freya, has been on a spiritual path for years. She realized her biggest dream was to have her own coaching business, so she could share her gifts and have location and financial freedom. However, for many years, she felt stuck in her regular job that didn't bring her joy. She felt like she didn't have the time or money to start her own business. And yet, she felt the longing in her heart becoming stronger and stronger. When Freya learned about the power of affirmations, she started to become aware of her negative self-talk. Surprisingly, she found that she constantly said to herself "I can't. I can't start a business. I can't be successful. I can't have financial freedom. It's just not possible for me." For so long, she wasn't aware that this was her constant self-talk. Whenever an opportunity presented itself, Freya would talk herself out of it. She reflected on her childhood and found that she was constantly told by her parents that she couldn't do what she wanted to do - "There isn't enough money. Life isn't a fairytale. You better be careful. Keep yourself small and please others so you can stay safe and lovable." These beliefs were ingrained into her being and stopped her from moving forward.

Freya started the journey of being aware of her beliefs and self-talk, and interrupting these patterns. Her new affirmations were: "There is always enough money to fulfill my heart's desires. I am supported in all that I do. I can only be successful. It is safe to be me and to be wealthy. I fully express myself. I am a successful business owner and financially free. I can create wealth by doing what I love and sharing my gifts and talents. I am capable of creating my dream life." At first.. nothing happened. After a few weeks, Freya noticed that she felt differently. Her automatic self-talk had changed and there were small changes in her environment. After a few months, she realized that naturally she had started sharing her gifts as a coach, and she celebrated having her first paying client. It didn't take long until her business made more money than her regular job, and she started going full-time. Today, she is working online, doing what she loves from anywhere in the world.

MAKE A DIFFERENCE WITH YOUR REVIEW!
Unlock the power of generosity...

> "Let the beauty of what you love be what you do. There
> are a thousand ways to kneel and kiss the ground."
> — *Rumi*

Hey there!

I do hope you have been enjoying, "The Art of Positive Affirmations &
Mantras: Harnessing the Power for Personal Growth and Fulfillment," by
B.M. Wolf. Your thoughts and opinions matter to me, and I'd love to hear
what you think about the book!

Your review can make a big difference. It not only helps fellow readers decide
if this book is right for them but also supports the author (me) in their
mission to spread the benefits of affirmations and mantras far and wide.

Remember, there are a thousand ways to kneel and kiss the ground; your
review has the power to touch lives beyond your own. So, why not take a
moment to share your thoughts and experiences with others?

Spread the joy of affirmations and mantras by leaving a review today. Together, let's unlock the power of generosity and make a positive impact in the world, one review at a time.

CHAPTER FIVE
EXPLORING SACRED MANTRAS FROM DIFFERENT TRADITIONS

> "The garden of the world has no limits, except in your mind."
> — *Rumi*

*C*hanting can be seen as negative overall depending on what culture you are from. In modern societies, mantras are often labeled as weird or scary, which hides their true power. In reality, chanting is not only part of many indigenous cultures but also part of Christianity with Gregorian chants. Movies and social media have twisted chanting to be often seen in horror or eclectic movies with a negative use. However, we now have science to help back up the benefits of chanting words or phrases. Some mantras even seem to have more benefits than others. Mantras can be seen as a tool to unlock the potential of the mind.

INTRODUCTION OF THE OM, GAYATRI, AND OM SO HUM MANTRA

When most people think of mantras, the first ones that come to mind are mantras related to Sanskrit, Hinduism, or Buddhism. While these philosophies have popularized mantras more into the mainstream, other cultures use mantras as a sacred practice as well. From the second largest Native American Nation, the Navajo, to the Aboriginal people of Australia, chanting mantras has always played an important role in all aspects of life;

from healing the sick to keeping the land alive and rich in resources. In Ancient Egypt, people practiced mantras to pray for an abundance of water in the Nile River, and in Shamanism, practitioners chant mantras to create deeper bonds with nature and to enhance connections in communities. [1] The practice of mantras in diverse cultural groups all over the world points to their significance and transformational power.

In today's world, you might recognize another use of mantras in the mainstream; when people get together at sports festivities, protests, or political events, they tend to chant a certain phrase repeatedly. This strengthens their coherence as a group, promotes teamwork, and achieves a common goal. Although this seems very different from chanting ancient Sanskrit mantras, they fulfill a similar purpose and show the power of mantras in our modern world. [2] Imagine people coming together at such a large scale, and chanting ancient, meaningful mantras for peace in the world!

The most famous mantra known for peace is the sacred mantra "Om". As we have already mentioned, the primordial sound of the Om Mantra is powerful and is now backed by scientific studies. Research shows that chanting om leads to coherence in the brain and has a calming effect, especially for those who experience chronic stress. [3] Studies have also demonstrated that there is a higher mental awareness in those who regularly chant Om; their physiology calms down, meaning more beneficial, slower respiration and blood pressure. It has also been shown that repetition of particular mantras, like Om, leads to the synchronicity of cardiovascular rhythms, suggesting it creates positive psychological and physiological effects. [4] Mantra has been shown to reduce psychological distress and improve mental health [5], although more research is needed. From my own point of view, mantras can help us through many distressful situations. Besides these measurable beneficial effects, symbolism has a strong meaning in spirituality and shamanism, something that science has difficulty interpreting. As we chant a mantra repeatedly, we can intuitively sense its symbolism and meaning, beyond what we can understand with our mind.

Another mantra of significance is the Gayatri mantra. My dear friend, Burma of *Wanderlust Malas and Reiki* [6] has a most beautiful practice of creating malas beads and infusing them with reiki while chanting the Gayatri mantra. It is such a beautiful practice and makes each mala so special. So what is the Gayatri mantra? Gayatri is a universal prayer to realize a higher state of consciousness. Translated, it means: "We meditate on pure consciousness, whose divine light illumines all realms. May this divine light illumine our intellect.' [7] The pure consciousness that we seek as the Divine is also within us. The Gayatri mantra helps us realize that the Divine light, consciousness, is the essence of all, and to remember ourselves as this essence: *"Now, the light which shines above in heaven, pervading all the spaces, pervading everywhere, both below and in the farthest reaches of the worlds—this indeed is that same light which shines within man."*—(*Chhandogya Upanishad 3.13.7*) [8]

Gayatri Mantra:
Om bhur, bhuvah, svah tat savitur varenyam bhargo devasya dhimahi dhiyo yo nah prachodayat

Om So Hum is another mantra, that is so simple yet elegant in nature. The mantra means, "I am that" and helps us to recognize the oneness in all things [9] It refers to *Atman*, the true self, divine consciousness in all forms. [10] This reminds me of Neil Walsh in his book, "Conversations with God." I watched him in an interview where he was talking about driving the street and seeing God and Self in everyone and everything and how liberating, beautiful, and comforting it is. There is also a beautiful quote: *"I've never seen anything other than the Divine, and neither did you."* What do you see when you walk, pedal, or drive down the street? What confronts you or causes your mind to judge? Homelessness? Addition? Obesity? Green Hair? Nose Piercings? Religious Groups? The Felon just released from Prison? Poverty? Wealth? Om So Hum! I am THAT! Each person, each sentient being is an embodiment of God. Can you see everything and everyone through the eyes of love? We all come from an infinite source. When this is adopted and applied, ultimately when we judge or criticize another we are judging and criticizing ourselves and the Divine. This mantra can also take on the following meanings: I am Love, I am abundance, I am acceptance, I am all that is good. "I am" refers to the Divine essence of everything. For some, knowing the meaning of the mantra can create a deeper connection with the phrase. For others, the proof is in the practice. The repetition. The routine. By deepening into ourselves as the Divine, mantra meditation has the power to transform the heart and the soul.

EXPLORING THE MEANINGS AND INTENTIONS BEHIND MANTRA AND KIRTAN KRIYA YOGA (MEDITATION) AND ITS UNIQUE BENEFITS

When sitting down to practice mantra meditation, it is good to set an intention or ask yourself questions to understand what mantra to chant. I started the practice of asking myself three sacred questions every morning about three years ago as suggested by my teacher, davidji, and it has helped me grow, revealed what I truly desired, and helped me with daily gratitude. The questions are:

1 - *Who am I when I'm at my best?*
2 - *Who and what am I grateful for?*
3 - *What does my heart truly long for?*

Sometimes I receive answers right away, sometimes I do not. Sometimes I get them later on in the day as my morning routine has prepared me to keep my heart and mind open to receiving. Another way to connect deeper with the mantra practice is to contemplate an intention you have for the day. Something simple, and achievable that you would like to see unfold today. It could be a specific outcome or a quality that you want to evoke. It shouldn't be too complicated. When you can see the intention clearly in your mind's eye, plant that intention deep within your nourishing heart center, and then let it go and move into your mantra meditation while trusting that your intention will be realized. [11]

It does not seem right to talk about mantras without mentioning this life-altering mantra, Kirtan Kriya Yoga. What is Kirtan Kriya Yoga meditation? It involves chanting sacred sounds, *Saa Taa Naa Maa* along with specific finger movements, mudras. Kirtan Kriya Yoga is associated with supernatural abilities in Tantric Buddhism called *siddhis*. It is said that if an aspirant practices for 2.5 hours daily for one year, they will develop knowledge of the unknowable, and start seeing the unseeable. [12] Most people in today's modern world will not be able to dedicate 2.5 hours in their busy days to mantra practice. However, it is known that practicing Kirtan Kriya Yoga for just 12 minutes a day can decrease stress in the body, enhance memory [13], improve general cognitive abilities, and prevent Alzheimer's disease. [14]

When I do group classes or teach this at the treatment center, people are amazed at everything this non-religious practice can do. This can be made into a spiritual practice or used for pure physical and mental benefits. I often hear statements such as, "I have a hard time meditating but this was easy and I had no chatter," or "I can see how this helps people meditate, I feel so good." This is a rhythmic and melodic chant that induces the traditional benefits of mantra and meditation but with an added cognitive bonus. Take a few minutes and give it a try.

Try it: Kirtan Kriya Yoga meditation practice

Assume a comfortable seating position with a straight spine, the hands resting on your body. Allow yourself to relax, and connect with your heart center.

Once you feel ready, start chanting the mantra *Saa, Taa, Naa, Maa*. With each sound, alternate through four hand gestures: [15]

1. On *Saa,* touch the first finger related to knowledge
2. On *Taa,* touch the second finger symbolizing wisdom, intelligence, and patience
3. On *Naa,* touch the third finger, associated with vitality, energy of life
4. On *Maa,* touch the fourth finger enhancing our ability to communicate

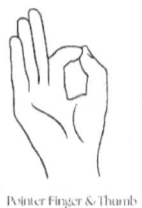
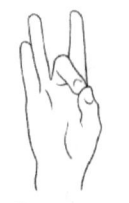
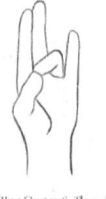
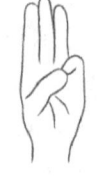

Pointer Finger & Thumb
Chin Mudra

Middle Finger & Thumb
Akash Mudra

Ring Finger & Thumb
Prithvi Mudra

Pinky Finger & Thumb
Varun Mudra

Images: Canva Pro

The practice alternates between chanting loudly, whispering, and in silence. For a 12-minute practice, begin by chanting the mantra out loud for 2 minutes. Then, continue chanting in a whisper for 2 minutes. Then, mentally repeat the mantra for 4 minutes. Then, again whisper the mantra for 2 minutes, and finally chant aloud for 2 minutes.[16]

You can also add a visualization if you like: [17]

"Each time you chant Saa, picture all the galaxies, planets, suns, moons, and stars.

Taa: visualize tremendous radiance, the brilliant, dazzling light of a trillion suns.

Naa: see a winter landscape, the branches of the barren trees standing silent in the snow, all of nature dormant.

Maa: picture thousands of spring flowers in a burst of glorious technicolor, brilliant blooms joyfully blanketing the hillside as far as the eye can see."

— *Shakti Parwha Kaur*

THE POTENCY OF A BUDDHIST MANTRA, OM MANI PADME HUM

Perhaps one of the most well-known Buddhist Mantras is Om Mani Padme Hum. It is the compassion mantra. "Thus, when a person who has recited ten malas of OM MANI PADME HUM a day goes into a river or an ocean, the water that touches the person's body gets blessed, and this blessed water then purifies all the billions and billions of sentient beings in the water. So it's unbelievably beneficial; this person saves the animals in that water from the most unbelievable suffering of the lower realms." [18] When translated it has an esoteric meaning of, "The Jewel is in the Lotus." This can be hard to understand as it does not have a direct translation to capture the full meaning. We will do our best here.

If we try to translate the mantra, it would be: " In order to reach enlightenment and obtain the pure mind, body, and speech of a Buddha, one must follow the path of dharma, a path built upon the inextricable union of wisdom and the Buddhist practices of compassion and love." [19]

Usually, in our daily lives, we are constantly distracted by the chatter of our minds. Our actions are usually based on egoic tendencies, based on anger, attachment, and ignorance. Thus, we create suffering for ourselves and others (although, ultimately, there are no others.) This is referred to as creating negative karma in Buddhism. [20] By chanting the Om Mani Padme Hum mantra, we go beyond the distractions of our mind; we open our minds and hearts to universal compassion, and thus we purify our karma. It is said that this practice ultimately leads to enlightenment. In Asian countries such as Tibet, Nepal, and India, there are retreats in which the mantra is recited 100 million times to alleviate the suffering in the world. [21] In these unprecedented times of suffering, war, and forgetfulness of our true nature on this planet, the practice of Om Mani Padme Hum is very powerful; even if just chanted for ten minutes during our daily practice.

Exercise:

Let's take a moment to feel the calmness and power of Om Mani Padme Hum. Take a long slow deep breath in through your nose and as you reach the top of your breath, ever so gently release your breath, just as slow.

Continue to watch your breath, and repeat the mantra once outloud, Om Mani Padme Hum; now repeat it as a whisper, Om Mani Padme Hum. Now repeat it silently to yourself for a few moments over and over while you gently close your eyes.

Remember, if you get distracted by thoughts, sounds, or physical sensations, just effortlessly come back to your mantra.

Once finished, let the stillness and silence settle in for a few moments while you witness and observe the calm and tranquility that, Om Mani Padme Hum, created. In just a few moments of repeating this mantra we have created space and raised the vibration.

CHAPTER SIX
AMPLIFYING RESULTS WITH VISUALIZATION AND MEDITATION

"What you seek is seeking you."
— *Rumi*

*W*e have learned about the magic of affirmations and how to choose them. We have also learned about the sacredness of mantras and the transformative power behind them. Now, we are going to put everything together to create a real transformation. How can we alchemize the use of mantras and affirmations in our daily lives and amplify the results?

ENHANCING THE EFFECTIVENESS OF AFFIRMATIONS THROUGH VISUALIZATION TECHNIQUES

Visualization is one of the most powerful tools to enhance the effectiveness of affirmations. It's an essential tool for helping our minds co-create with the universe. If you have goals you would like to manifest, visualizing the end result every day kicks your manifestation into full gear. Visualization means that you create a vivid mental image of your desired outcome in your mind. You visualize your desired outcome as if it is already a reality; you use all your senses to see, hear, smell, taste, and touch it. In this way, you are programming your subconscious mind to draw your desire to you. Your subconscious mind can't differentiate between what you imagine as real and what is already a reality. Therefore, if you imagine and feel your desire to be a reality now, your subconscious mind will work towards its fulfillment. [1] If we look at it from a more scientific perspective, by visualizing your goals, you create new neural pathways in your brain, which are similar to the ones created if you were experiencing your desires in physical reality already. [2] As such, combining visualization with affirmations can be seen as an "inner highway" toward your desires.

Some people find visualization challenging. They often say, "I can meditate, but I cannot visualize." That's okay; it's a practice, not perfection. You can choose from many different visualization techniques, and we will now explore the most powerful ones.

DAILY VISUALIZATION

The most common visualization technique is to visualize your desired outcome for two minutes twice a day, just after waking up and just before going to bed with your eyes closed. You can visualize your desire in any way that feels natural to you. Some guiding questions can be: How would you see the world if your desire was already a reality? What would you see, hear, taste, and touch? Where would you be? How would you feel? If you find it difficult to visualize, you can play some inspiring music that uplifts you and helps you go within. When visualizing your desires, make sure that you truly feel the joy, excitement, and gratitude for your desire being a reality. These elevated emotions help draw your desire to you.

YOUR DESIRE AS A MOVIE SCENE

A very powerful, related manifestation technique is to decide on one scene that would happen if your desire was a reality. The scene can last anywhere between 5 and 15 seconds. For example, if you are manifesting a romantic connection, your scene could be on a beach at sunset, looking into the eyes of your partner and feeling them holding your hands. If you are manifesting financial abundance, the scene could be that you see more money coming into your bank account, and you beautifully invest the money. When choosing a scene, make sure it feels natural to you and that visualizing the scene makes you feel great. Once you decide on a scene, every evening just before going to bed, keep playing that scene over and over again in your mind until you fall asleep while feeling grateful for your desire already being a reality. This ensures that you fall asleep in your desired reality, and your subconscious mind will be deeply imprinted during your sleep.

ROLE PLAY

If you find it challenging to visualize in your mind's eye, this technique might be for you. For a few moments, contemplate who you would be if your desire was already a reality. How would that person feel, think and behave? How would they walk around? How do they engage with the world? Write out a description of this person as if you were creating a character for a role play. Include the feelings, thoughts, and behaviors of that person. Now, you get to have fun! Choose one day and commit to embodying that person. It might feel very uncomfortable at first as you are used to your old ways of being; however, these old ways got you to where you are now. If you want to create change, you have to create a new way of being, even if it feels uncomfortable. Don't forget that your system is hard-wired to keep you safe to survive, not to create your desires and live your dream life. In short, think, feel, and act like the person who already lives in the reality of your desire, and watch how quickly your life will change!

INNER DIALOGUE

This creative visualization technique is often overlooked but very powerful. We all talk to ourselves internally most of the day. We have an ongoing inner dialogue, although most of the time, we are not aware of it. Most of us have an inner dialogue that keeps perpetuating our current reality, for example: "There are no good men out there. I will never find a partner." or "And again, I am broke. I can't afford anything." or "I just can't change. I'm stuck." Sounds familiar? With the inner dialogue technique, you will let go of the familiar, negative inner dialogue and create a new, empowering dialogue aligned with your desire. If your desired outcome was already a reality, how would you speak to yourself? For example, if you were in a fulfilling romantic relationship, possibly you would say: "Wow, I feel so loved. There is so much romance in my life." If you were financially abundant, you might say to yourself: "I love feeling so wealthy and having more than enough money to sustain myself." Write down both the old dialogue and the new dialogue. Then, for a few minutes of a day, for example, when you are having lunch by yourself, start practicing this new inner dialogue. Speak to yourself as if your desire was already a reality. It might feel unfamiliar at first, but the more you practice, the more natural it will become.

GRATITUDE

This might not sound like a visualization technique, but it's very close. For this practice, below or in a notebook, write down five things you are grateful for in your current life, as well as five things from the future you are grateful for. Write all statements in the present tense, even if some of them haven't happened yet. For example, if you are manifesting a romantic relationship, you could write: "I am so grateful that I met my beautiful partner, and I love living life with him/her." If you are manifesting financial abundance, one of your statements could be: "I am so grateful for all the money in my bank account. It feels wonderful to know there is always enough money." It is essential for this exercise to feel the gratitude in your heart.

_____

_____

_____

_____

_____

_____

_____

_____

SCRIPTING

Still not convinced that visualization is for you? This technique can be practiced without any mental imagery. Below or in a notebook, write the date one year from now. Assume that it is one year from now, and your manifestation has become a reality. Then, write down what the life of the version of you looks like that already lives in your desired reality. What does their day look like? Where do they live? What do they do? What's the number on their bank account? Write the description from your perspective in the present tense, and include how you feel. For example "It feels amazing that I have a successful online business and work from my beach house."

_____

_____

_____

_____

_____

_____

_____

_____

_____

_____

_____

_____

_____

_____

_____

_____

_____

_____

_____

_____

_____

_____

_____

_____

_____

_____

_____

THE HEART OF VISUALIZATION

When visualizing, it is important to surrender and not to have expectations. I know I know...but how do you not have expectations when you are creating something? It's more of letting go of the "cursed hows." You clearly visualize the end result, and you let go of any hows. How is this going to come to fruition? Which way will it happen? When we visualize, we want to see it as if it has already happened. We do not want to visualize the journey there - the universe will handle that. We want to see it as if it is done and complete. In that way, yes you can expect the final result however it may look. Just not the minutiae of "how" it came to be. Isn't that liberating? You don't have to know how your manifestation will come to you. If you knew how you would most likely already be doing it. By visualizing the end result, we set forces into motion that are beyond our understanding. These forces are universal in nature - some call this invisible force universal intelligence or the Divine. By being at the vibration of your desire (you already achieved it), you allow the Universe to organize people, places, and things to serve your desire and to bring it into physical reality.

If you are creating a new way to earn money, visualize yourself creating wealth, feeling the feeling of being there, and seeing what it might look like without putting in the hows. If you are a single mom looking to go to the grocery store and shop without a budget, see yourself buying organic foods, purchasing what you want without always shopping for cheap brands or looking at the prices. See yourself buying the brand you want paying for your groceries and leaving the store happy with the feeling of having more money in your wallet. By the way, that was me. Manifesting an expanded budget for groceries was very important to me. At one point in my life, our main food was peanut butter, bread, ramen, and eggs and we were having garage sales to pay rent. It was just what it was at the time. We were lucky to live in a rental, but I heavily relied on the school lunch program to feed my daughter, my job, and the one free meal I got to take home per shift. My daughter and I would often split it. I wanted to buy my daughter what she wanted, feed her healthy options, and not feel stressed when I left the store. Affirmations and visualization became a daily part of my life. "I buy whatever we like at the grocery store, and there is money to spare." "My grocery budget is expansive, and there is always enough." When I was going to the store, I would visualize myself being able to buy more, and if it was within my budget to buy something extra, I would! On the way out of the store, I would practice gratitude for being able to buy everything we needed and desired. "Thank you thank you thank you for my expansive grocery budget." To this day, my daughter will no longer eat peanut butter. These affirmations and visualizations helped me manifest more quickly. Unexpected money came several times during this period until finally, I accepted a job offer that I could support us with. It was so freeing to walk into the grocery store and pass the peanut butter and the ramen. But, at the time, I didn't know how this financial freedom would manifest. I kept visualizing and affirming it, trusting that the universe would find the most beneficial way.

DEEPEN MEDITATION WITH INTENTION AND MANTRAS

How do we go deeper in mediation? There are many ways to do this, but for this book, we are setting intentions and using mantras as our "mind vehicles" to assist us in going deeper. Mantra partnered with intention is where the Self can be found. This means listening to your heart and finding out what your heart truly longs for. Then, set an intention to let your heart's desires unfold within your life. An intention is defined as "a directed thought to perform a determined action". [3] Our intentions seem to operate as highly coherent frequencies capable of changing the molecular structure of matter. [4] Intent may not seem like it is that big of a deal, however, we now have studies to prove otherwise. Thanks to the findings of Dr. Emoto, we know that positive intent has the power to form beautiful crystals within ice and negative intent has the power to create more erratic shapes in frozen ice. [5] Since we are 70% water, the power of intention has an impact on us as well. Prior to meditating, getting a clear vision of something you would like to see unfold throughout the day or possibly something larger you are working towards can help align yourself with the end result.

So, let's get into the exact process of how to deepen meditation with intention and mantras. Start by finding a comfortable seated position, and take some deep breaths in and out. Then, start breathing into your heart center, which is located in the middle of the chest, a little to the right. Allow your heart to gently open. Then, feel into your heart and let it express what it truly longs for. Listen to the whispers of your heart. Once you have received a desire from your heart, let it blossom into an intention. While staying connected to your heart center, commit to the intention to let your heart's desire unfold in your life. Plant it deeply within your heart. Take a few moments to clearly visualize your heart's desire in your mind's eye, seeing it as if it was already reality. Deepen into the trust that this desire is already yours; that it will happen for you. Choose a mantra that aligns with your intention (see Chapter 8 for an extensive list) and move into mantra meditation, either with or without a mala. Get a feel for the mantra by saying it out loud once, whispering it once, and then repeating it silently over and over. If you get distracted by thoughts, sounds, or physical sensations, don't worry. Easily and effortlessly, come back to your mantra and your breath. The more you come back to your mantra and breathe, the easier it is to entrain your mind and keep your focus on the present. Then, as you go about your day, stay connected to the intention you planted into your heart center.

THE POWER OF VISUALIZATION AND MITATION IN MANIFESTING GOALS

A family member of mine has become increasingly more powerful in manifesting things within her own life. Most recently, she manifested $6400 to pay off the remaining balance of her car. How did she do this? Several ways - on her vision board, she had a reminder that her car was paid off already. She owned it free and clear, as if it had already happened, staying away from the details of "how" it happened. When she would get into her car, she would say out loud with feeling, "Thank you thank you thank you Universe, I am so happy my car is paid for in full. Yes! Yes! Yes!" She did this with unwavering faith that she knew something would come through. Every time she made a payment, she would thank the Universe again and feel the feeling. She would visualize herself driving down the road in a paid-for car. How do you visualize this? By quite literally "getting the feels"! What would it feel like to have your desire happen? One day, another family member called with the good news of some unexpected money that he was sharing with her and that he had already put a cheque in the mail for $6400. She received the cheque a few days later and thanked the Universe on the way to the bank to pay off her car. Her unwavering practice of her affirmation and gratitude along with visualizing her car being paid for and feeling that emotion ultimately attracted the money to her. This is the power of changing our state of being and living as if our desire was already a reality!

CHAPTER SEVEN
AFFIRMATION STATION

> "You are not a drop in the ocean. You are the entire
> ocean in a drop."
> — *Rumi*

*A*s you look through this next chapter, mark which affirmations are for you; put a check or a star next to the ones that really resonate with you. There will be a space for you to write down some of your own or list your favorites. We will begin by having a look at mirror work, a transformative way to practice your affirmations. Then, we will explore an abundance of affirmations.

MIRROR WORK

To level this affirmation process up, and to make the most of the affirmations you choose, consider saying your affirmations in front of a mirror. A mirror doesn't only reflect your outer physical image but also the inner image you have of yourself. It reflects where you resist fully loving and accepting yourself and which affirmations make you feel open and loving. [1] Saying affirmations to yourself in the mirror is a powerful tool that shows you precisely the thoughts and beliefs about yourself that you need to change to transform your life. When you first start doing mirror work, there will likely be a lot of resistance. After all, we have never learned to truly love who we are, let alone to say "I love you" to ourselves in the mirror. One of my students told me that the first time she did mirror work, everything in her was resisting, and she immediately wanted to stop. However, there is a lot of wisdom in the resistance, and if we can soften, even a little bit, and keep going, our lives will inevitably change. It is recommended to practice mirror work for at least 21 consecutive days when you first get started.

Try it: A step-by-step guide to starting your mirror work journey.

1. For the first time, you do mirror work, and for 2-3 minutes at the beginning of each session, practice being present and looking into your eyes. While focusing on one eye, start seeing and feeling the love in you. Beyond all the conditioning, the resistance, the frustration, the unwanted habits... See the love that you are in your essence. It might not be easy at first, but as you keep practicing, you will start to feel a softening and openness. It can be helpful to center in your heart when you engage in this practice.

2. Start with affirmations that you feel in resonance with, that feels good to you, and that you love saying. They should feel uplifting and not evoke too much resistance. If you can't think of any affirmation that makes you feel good, think of past successes or anything you are proud of or grateful for.

3. Then, practice all of your chosen affirmations by saying them to yourself in the mirror. When resistance comes up, allow it to be there. Let it guide you to the places within yourself that you now get to love.

4. Conclude your practice with a moment of gratitude and connect with your heart. Allow any feelings to be there, and breathe deeply into them.

5. Continue this process for at least 21 days. It can take time to get over the initial barriers; therefore it is called mirror *work*; it truly is a journey. [2]

UNIVERSAL AFFIRMATIONS

The following affirmations are inspired by "The Four Agreements" by Don Miguel Ruiz.

- I am impeccable with my word.
- I know that what others do is about them, not me.

- I say what I mean and ask others questions in order to have clear communication.
- I always do my best.

AFFIRMATIONS FOR SELF-LOVE AND ACCEPTANCE

This can be a sensitive topic for many, as past wounds can bury themselves deep within our bodies and physiology. Even after we have let them go, they can leave us feeling unloved, unaccepted, and unwanted. The past is the past; you are an adult now, and you have the power to create the love, acceptance, and desire you need all within your heart.

- With every breath, I am new.
- Today and every day I am loved.
- I wholeheartedly accept myself and others.
- I am a good person and make choices for the highest and best good.
- Myself and others are beautiful, kind, and loving.
- I express the best version of myself daily.
- I accept and embrace my imperfections.
- I am kind to my human side.
- My body is beautiful in every way.
- I am strong and accept challenges with a brave heart.
- I love myself.
- I am a magnificent being.
- I am a spiritual being in a human body.
- I love who I am, and who I am becoming.
- I am worthy, just by existing.
- I was born worthy of love.
- I am a divine expression of the universe.
- My true essence is love.
- I am wonderful, just the way I am.
- My greatest success is being me, unapologetically.
- I am beautiful, just by being me.

- I am loving towards myself and others.
- I am the priority. I care for my well-being.
- I fully choose and love myself.
- I am unique and perfect as I am.
- I deeply trust myself.
- I am a gift to this world.
- My presence is a blessing to the world.
- I fully allow myself to express who I really am.
- Loving myself allows me to live in the greatest expression of myself.
- I fill myself up with love and kindness.
- I am stable and secure within myself.
- I have a gentle, loving heart.
- It's easy for me to be me.
- Everything I need is within me.
- I know I am powerful.
- I see the power in me.
- I live in surrender to my heart.
- I am forever conscious of my true worth.

HEALTH AND WELL-BEING

- All of my 50 trillion cells are working together at an optimal level for my highest and best good.
- My immune system is strong and works on my behalf to remain healthy.
- I am mentally, emotionally, and physically sound.
- It feels good to take care of my body.
- My powerful body knows how to heal itself.
- With every breath, my body heals.
- I give myself permission to find joy and experience pleasure.
- I forgive myself and others and am free of the past.
- I know my worth and expect only goodness.
- It's okay for negative emotions to arise, as they will also pass.

- Every cell of my being is filled with love.
- I trust the wisdom of my body.
- I treat my body like a sacred temple.
- I honor the whispers of my body.
- I love all parts of my body.
- I allow myself to feel vital and alive.
- My health is getting better and better every day.
- I love treating my body with love.
- I rest when my body asks for it.
- I live in alignment with the cycles of my body.

SUCCESS AND ACHIEVEMENT

- I am surrounded by inspiration.
- I am courageous in my pursuit of success.
- I have a purpose and inspire others.
- I take time to play and relax as it aids in my success.
- Challenges help me grow and see something for myself.
- I am the co-creator of my life.
- I let my heart lead the way.
- My success plan includes the success of others.
- When I help another, I know I'm on the right path.
- I celebrate my achievements with love.
- I am devoted to unfolding my full potential.
- I embrace and love my success.
- I live my life to the fullest.
- I love taking action on my dreams.
- I have meaning and purpose for being here.
- I am a magnet for success.
- I am capable of creating extraordinary success.
- It's easy for me to live my destiny.
- I live my true soul's purpose.

- Every day, I deepen into an expression of my soul's purpose.
- Life is always happening for me, not to me.
- I am on the perfect journey to my success.
- My journey to success is unique and unfolding in divine timing.
- All potentials exist for me right now.
- I am the creator of my life.
- I deeply trust myself.
- I believe in myself and my potential.

ABUNDANCE AND PROSPERITY

- I am financially free.
- Money is energy that enhances my life experiences.
- When I spend money, I circulate abundance.
- I am financially free, location free, and time free.
- My personal abundance and prosperity are in alignment with who I am.
- Abundance is my birthright.
- I thrive. I am a thriver.
- I am a money magnet.
- As if by magic, the money is always there.
- I am in vibrational alignment with abundance.
- I have more than enough to support my lifestyle, investments, gifting, and fun.
- I get to have all the money in the world.
- I deserve extraordinary wealth.
- The more money I have, the better it is for the world.
- Through money, my generous heart has ways to express itself.
- Money amplifies my goodness.
- I can be spiritual and wealthy.
- I believe in limitless abundance.
- I know I exist in a world of limitless abundance.
- I am wealthy doing what I love.

- I create my level of wealth.
- There is always enough because I am enough.
- Everything I desire flows to me easily.
- I love money, and money loves me.
- I am prosperity
- I like money, I love it, I use it wisely.
- Money is constantly circulating in my life.
- I release money with joy, and it returns to me multiplied.
- Money flows to me in abundance.
- I am grateful for the riches of my mind.
- It is my right to be rich, happy, and successful.
- My abundance is in alignment with integrity.

GRATITUDE AND APPRECIATION

- I am grateful for every life lesson, celebration, and moment of joy.
- I know my life is not possible without the help of others, and I'm grateful.
- Who I am today is a reflection of yesterday, thank you.
- I am in awe and grateful for every sunrise.
- I am most grateful for the simple things.
- Gratitude, love, and compassion fill my soul.
- Gratitude is the healing balm that binds us together.
- I appreciate the kindness in others that is reflected within me.
- I appreciate the grace that has been given to me.
- Gratitude and appreciation give me a new perspective.
- I am grateful for being me.
- I am grateful for all the little daily moments of joy and connection.
- I feel grateful for each part of my being.
- Every morning, I rise in gratitude.
- I am grateful for the magic of this universe.
- I am grateful for life.

HAPPINESS AND JOY

- I vibe high, and everywhere I go, the vibration is raised.
- Joy and happiness happen with ease.
- I cultivate a beautiful life free from negative thinking.
- I am aligned and attract happiness and joy.
- I'm at peace with my past and joyful in the present moment.
- I have unlimited joy, abundance, and prosperity.
- I move forward in life with happiness.
- I accomplish the mundane with ease and presence.
- I inhale joy and exhale anxiety.
- Positive energy moves through every aspect of my life.
- I love embracing my joy and pleasure.
- It is safe for me to feel good.
- By expressing my joy, others feel joy, too.
- I am deeply aligned with the joy of being alive.
- My happiness is an inner state and only depends on me.
- I choose to live my life with joy.

RELATIONSHIPS AND CONNECTION

- My gratitude for love runs deep.
- Me and partner are living our best lives together.
- I am surrounded by others who love me and cheer me on.
- I give, I love, I receive, and do it again.
- Authentic love stems from me.
- I see love and connection everywhere I go.
- Love comes easily to me.
- I am smart, kind, and have much to offer.
- I trust and have an open heart.
- My partner and I have love, commitment, and trust for each other.
- Access to me is sacred.
- It is safe for me to love and be loved.

- I am in alignment with unconditional love.
- Others love being around me.
- I am worthy of being chosen and prioritized.
- I reveal my authentic self in connections with others.
- I always stay connected to my heart.
- I see others through the eyes of love.
- I see the Divine in my partner.
- Others support me in creating my dream life, and I support others.
- I am supported in all that I do.
- I deeply love myself and others.

SPIRITUALITY AND INNER PEACE

- I receive and am grateful for all the abundance the universe gives me.
- My thoughts bring the highest and best good into my life.
- I trust the divine timing of the universe.
- I let go and trust.
- The peace within me is reflected in the world around me.
- I open my heart and receive divine inspiration.
- I use my unique talents and gifts to contribute to society and help others.
- It is more important for me to invoke peace rather than duality.
- I'm ok with how others choose to live their life.
- I can handle any situation.
- My mind is open to new possibilities.
- The universe is limitless, and so am I.
- I deeply trust myself and life.
- I am safe to let go and receive.
- Everything I desire is on its way to me.
- I love allowing my desires to come to me.
- I am an embodiment of love and peace.
- I am deeply at peace with myself and life.
- Every obstacle turns into an opportunity.

- I learn and grow every day.
- I love to align deeper and deeper with the universe.
- I am deeply connected to universal intelligence.
- I love embodying my higher self.
- I am always divinely guided in all that I do.
- I act from presence and love.

Now, let's take a few moments to write down which affirmations resonate with you the most. Possibly, you might enjoy blending a few to create something unique for your life. Remember to speak as if it is already here without the details of how it happens. For example, if you are trying to manifest money, do not include details of how you get it or how it comes to be part of the affirmations. The universe handles the details. Above all else, focus on how the affirmation makes you feel. If you feel an openness in your heart, excitement, and a sense of joy, you have found the right affirmation for you. Make sure to also include affirmations of your desired manifestations that you currently feel in resistance with, as transforming the resistance will draw your manifestation to you. Don't overthink the process of choosing your affirmations; let it be intuitive. Trust yourself, have fun, and enjoy the process!

_____

_____

_____

_____

_____

_____

_____

_____

CHAPTER EIGHT
MINDFUL MANTRA MOMENTS

> "Absorbed in this world you've made it your burden.
> Rise above the world. There is another vision."
> — *Rumi*

*T*ake *your meditation deeper with mantras and let them weave their way into your life. This "mind-vehicle" with help you detach from the chatter, bring yourself to the present moment, de-escalate stress and anxiety, and raise your vibration. Each mantra has a brief description of what it means; you may recognize some from earlier in the book. Remember, you can use a mala with mantras for Japa Meditation.*

In this chapter, we are attempting to categorize mantras based on their meaning. However, mantras are interchangeable and often have a unique meaning that can't be put into words. Although the mantras are categorized, once you read the meaning, take it a step further and get to know the mantra for yourself. Then, you will find that they can fit into multiple categories. Still, for reference and to make it easier for our Western minds, categories seem to make sense.

Some of the mantras work well when they are used with mudras. *Mudra* means "gesture" in Sanskrit. Mudras were used in ancient yogic systems to allow life force energy to flow through us in specific, meaningful ways. The finger gestures can be seen as energetic circuits that enhance the flow of energy and thus intensify the practice of a mantra. Below, you will find an illustration of four common mudras, which can be used with several mantras listed below.

FOR SPIRITUAL GROWTH/LIBERATION

- *Om So Hum* (**Oneness/Acceptance**):

Translation - "I am That"

To connect with the universe, regulate your breathing, and soothe your mind. That is the main vibration of this mantra. We are recognizing that everything we see is somehow a reflection of ourselves. It's the ultimate in recognizing the oneness in all things.

- *Om Namah Shivaya (Consciousness):*

Translation - "I bow to the inner Self/Pure Consciousness/Shiva".

A famous Hindu mantra evoking pure consciousness.

- *Sat Chit Ananda (Limitlessness/Consciousness):*

Translation - "Sat - Existence, Chit (Cit) = Consciousness/Awareness, Ananda - Limitlessness."

Ananda can also mean bliss or joy. The mantra is for limitless conscious power. When tapping into the vibration of this mantra, it aligns us with the divine consciousness and brings about inner peace, joyfulness, and transcendence.

- *Ganesha Sharanam, Sharanam Ganesha (Refuge, Protection):*

Translation - "Surrender to the lotus feet of Lord Ganesha, Sharanum - Refuge/Protection/Sanctuary."

Ganesha is the elephant-headed son of Shiva and Parvati. Ganesha is considered to be the remover of obstacles. There are beautiful devotional songs dedicated to the mantra meaning. This mantra invokes the refuge of protection from Lord Ganesha.

- *This too, shall pass (Acceptance):*

  Acceptance of the moment and knowing that whether we perceive something as good, bad, chaotic, calm, happy, or sad, this moment right now will pass. Honor the moment and honor this feeling as, "This too, shall pass."

  This is great to use with mudras and match each word with a touch. First pointer to the thumb (this), middle to the thumb (too), ring to the thumb (shall), pinky to the thumb (pass). See illustration.

- *I am love (Unconditional Love):*

  This simple mantra is very powerful. It can help you reconnect with the love within yourself, and the universal love within all. It reminds you of your true nature if you tap into its meaning beyond thoughts. A variation of this mantra is "**My essential nature is love.**"

FOR FORGIVENESS AND COMPASSION

- *Om Mani Padme Hum (Enlightenment):*

  Translation - "Praise to the jewel in the lotus."

  This is known as the compassion mantra, "On the path of life, with intention and wisdom, we can achieve the pure body, speech, and mind of a Buddha." There is a saying that after practicing, "Om Mani Padme Hum," ten times on a mala, our vibration is high enough that if we touch water it will raise the vibration of all that is within the water.

- *Lokah Samastah Sukhino Bhavantu (Compassion):*

  Translation - "May all beings everywhere be happy and free," (short version). "May all beings everywhere be happy and free and may the thoughts, words, and actions of my own life contribute in some way to that happiness and to that freedom for all," (long version).

It's a mantra to dissolve the ego self and radiate positive energy to all beings. Be sure to include yourself in the part about "all beings." May you *also* be happy and free.

- *Ho'opono Opono (Reconcilliation):*

Translation - "I'm Sorry. Please Forgive Me. Thank you. I Love You."

An ancient Hawaiian mantra and the ultimate form of reconciliation. What is so beautiful about this is that it does not matter who is right and who is wrong, the reconciliation is more important. Taking responsibility for our own role, no matter what our part to play has been, whether we feel justified or not.

As an adult, we have the opportunity to recognize that we can not control things that happened to us as a child, and choose to not let them define our life. We have a choice to do things differently than how we were raised. We have a choice to let go of the story of "what happened" to us. We have a choice to heal from the pain and move on in life.

This mantra works well with the illustrated mudras. First pointer to the thumb (I'm sorry), middle to the thumb (please forgive me), ring to the thumb (thank you), pinky to the thumb (I love you). See photo.

TO HEAL PAIN AND SUFFERING AND REGULATE EMOTIONS

- *Tayata Om Bekandze Bekandze (Healing):*

Translation - "May the many sentient beings who are sick, be freed from sickness soon. And may all the sicknesses of beings never arise again."

It's known as the Medicine Buddha mantra and heals pain and suffering.

- *Om Moksha Ritam (Emotional Freedom):*

Translation - "Om, Emotional Freedom, Rhythm of the Universe."

The mantra for self-liberation. Om - Oneness of all, Moksha - Emotional Freedom, Ritam - Rhythm of the Universe. A mantra that calibrates oneself to that rhythm releasing us from the confines of conditioning.

- *Ananda Maya Moksha (Inner Healing):*

Translation - "Ananda can be limitlessness/joy/bliss, Maya is Illusion, Moksha is Emotional Freedom."

Liberating ourselves from negative thinking. Surrender to the power of our healing. Maya - Illusion. Negative thought patterns that cause us suffering are an illusion. Self-suffering is an illusion overall as we can choose to label our experiences or practice acceptance. The more we practice acceptance and let go of control, the more free we become.

- *I Can Handle This (Strength):*

As humans, we have some vast emotions. This is a mantra that can be used to aid in helping us reach a new grand goal that we set, overcome adversity or anxiety, and at times, get through the moment. "I can handle this," aids in in harnessing our inner strength and bringing it to the forefront of our life.

This mantra also works in conjunction with the illustrated mantra. Just like the previous mantra, touch each word with a finger. First pointer to the thumb (I), middle to the thumb (can), ring to the thumb (handle), pinky to the thumb (this). See mudra chart.

As a sidenote, mantras can have multiple meanings especially when translated. Sanskrit is a dead language and although scholars have done the very best they can, not all words can be translated easily into another language. A perfect example of this is, "Om Mani Padme Hum."

FOR ABUNDANCE AND PROSPERITY

- *Mahalakshmi Ashtakam (Wealth and gain):*

Translation - "Reverential Salutations to Lakshmi."

This mantra invokes the blessings of the Divine Mother, Lakshmi, and to have a prosperous and peaceful life. Ashtakam is a particular kind of poetry written in eight verses. Practicing this mantra is tapping into the vibration of prosperity which can present in many ways.

- *Om Hrim Shrim Lakshmi Bhyo Namaha (positivity and abundance, material and spiritual riches):*

Translation - "Goddess Lakshmi resides in me and bless me with your abundance in all spheres of my life."

You may have already recognized Lakshmi in this mantra. It is another great mantra dedicated to the Goddess Lakshmi. Wealth, prosperity, and abundance are symbiotic with Lakshi and when using this mantra it is inviting spiritual and material abundance into our lives.

OTHER BEAUTIFUL MANTRAS YOU MIGHT WANT TO EXPLORE

- *Om Mahasaraswate Namaha (Intellectual growth and creative expression):*

Translation: "Salutations to Saraswati."

This mantra is bringing guidance and inspiration into our lives. It connects us to the loving power of the Hindu Goddess *Saraswati*, and evokes her creativity. Traditionally, Saraswati is honored for her divine knowledge and wisdom.

- *Om Eim Saraswati Namaha Om (Awaken):*

Translation: "We call in Saraswati, the goddess of creativity and language."

This mantra is amazing for beginning creative projects. The sanskrit word, Eim (sounds like I'm) is the seed sound for the goddess Saraswati and invokes all that she stands for. She embodies Shakti energy in the form of creativity, language, wisdom, art, knowledge, and music.

- ***Om Hum Hanumate Namaha (courage, strength, and devotion):***

Translation: "Om and salutations to Hanuman, the embodiment of pure devotion. May I be blessed with victory, success, strength, stamina, and power."

The Hanuman Mantra evokes courage, inner strength, power, and physical strength. It is chanted in devotion to the Hindu God Hanuman, shaped as half monkey and half human. Hanuman helps us to fearlessly use our gifts to connect to the Divine through loving service and devotion.

"When I do not know who I am, I serve you. When I do know who I am, You and I are One." - Hanuman

- ***Metta (Compassion):***

Translation: "Unconditional loving - kindness."

This is known as the loving-kindness meditation. A mantra that allows us to send loving-kindness to those we know and love, and do not know, and stretch it to the far reaches of the cosmos. Metta is a compassion builder as we send more loving-kindness to others, the compassion in our heart grows. A client of mine shared with me, "When you pray for someone, you really grow to love them." She had been sharing a story of how she met and fell in love with her husband. It all started with sending loving-kindness in the form of prayer. That is the power of sending it out all people, even those we do not see alignment with, those that we may have a grudge or grievance with, and those we do not even know exist.

- ***Gate Gate Paragate Parasamgate Bodhi Svaha (Enlightenment):***

Translation: "Gone, gone, gone beyond, gone utterly beyond, Enlightenment, hail!"

There is so much wisdom in this mantra that an entire chapter could be dedicated to just this. I will do my best. It represents the wisdom around ancient sutras, "The Heart Sutra," and "The Diamond Sutra." As we chant this mantra, we are moving towards Oneness and away from separation. Letting go of duality. It reminds me of Ram Das in his pursuit of "Becoming Nobody." Letting go of who we are, the things that we identify with like eye color, hair color, our titles, and anything that may separate us from our One true essence.

- *Om Tare Tuttare Ture Svaha (Help, Strength, Compassion, Healing):*

Translation: "I prostrate to the Liberator, Mother of all the Victorious Ones."

Green Tara is often depicted as a compassionate goddess willing to offer protection and comfort from all the suffering in the world. Chanting this mantra has a lot of meaning behind it, and could be considered an advanced mantra by some. The following is a consolidated version to give an idea of the depth this mantra has. Chanting this mantra liberates one from the eight dangers: ignorance, anger, attachment, jealousy, pride, miserliness, doubt, and wrong views. It also frees one from the cause of suffering, that may not be so obvious. This mantra liberates one from disease and the true cause of disturbing thoughts.

If this mantra resonates with you, or if you find yourself interested in Green Tara, do more research on her and western minds do not grasp layers as easily. She is a beloved figure across the world.

- *Sat Nam Rasayan (Oneness):*

Translation: "Healing through the name/ "Abandonding oneself to the essence of pure Identity"

This mantra allows us to experience the deep tranquality of the mind, and to transcend ordinary consciousness for deep transcendental experiences. Ultimately, we deepen into our true nature, Oneness.

- *Om Shanti, Shanti, Shanti (Peace):*

Translation - "Om, Peace, Peace, Peace."

Shanti not only means something precious, it is also beautiful to say. When repeated three times it embodies peace in body, in speech and in mind. This is a great mantra to invoke peace both within yourself and when sending to others.

- **Ong Namo Guru Dev Namo (Bow to the teacher within, honoring thyself):**

    Translation: "I bow to the divine wisdom within myself."

    In a world that constantly wants us to seek wisdom and validation without, this mantra guides us back within to our wisdom. The mantra connects us to our inner guru, to trust ourselves and our innate wisdom, and it reminds us that we are our own best teachers. It also reminds us of our Divine essence, which is the same essence that's within all.

- **Om (Hymm of the Universe):**

    Translation: "Om."

    They hymn of the Universe. Like we discussed earlier, Om can be used over and over again to invoke a sense of calm and a sense of piece. Revisit chapter three for a refresher.

- **Ganesh Mantra: Om Gum Ganapatayei Namah (Remover of Obstacles):**

    Translation: "My salutations to Lord Ganesha."

    This mantra evoked the Hindu God Ganesha, known as the remover of obstacles and the grantor of success. Ganesha is depicted as an elephant-headed God, and very popular world-wide. Many practitioners chant this mantra to remove any obstacles they might face on their path.

- **Agne Meele Purhohitam (Transformation):**

    Translation: "I surrender to the fire of transformation."

    A mantra perfect for the many times in our life when growth and change presents itself. When we are shedding the old ways that no longer serve us and we invoke the power of Agni (fire) to burn away the remnants and transform into a better version of ourselves. I have used this mantra many times and have found tremendous value in, "Agne Meele Purohitam."

- *Lam, Vam, Ram, Yam, Ham, Sham, Om (Chakras):*

Translation: N/A

These are vibrations of the chakras, and therefore have no literal translation. When we chant these mantras, Lam (root), Vam (sacral), Ram (solar plexus), Yam (heart), Ham (throat), Sham (third eye), Om (crown), it vibrationally aligns our mantras. These work well outloud. When you chant them, your vagus nerve is stimulated and the vibration is now working through your energy centers. If there are two chakras you are working on aligning, like the root and the solar plexus, then you can chant, "Lam," and "Ram." Or, let's say it is the heart and third eye, "Yam," and "Sham." It is really up to you. A recommendation would be to practice the full vibrations together for a few minutes before transitioning into the specific chakras you are focused on.

- *Yoga Chitta Vritti Nirodha (Acceptance/Expanssion):*

Translation: "Yoga is the cessation of the fluctuations of the mind."

This mantra is stated in the famous yoga sutras of Patanjali (Sutra 1, Verse 2). It means that usually, we ignore the truth of our being, as we are lost in the fluctuations of the mind - thoughts and sensations. However, if we learn to stop identifying with these fluctuations, then we will find the true meaning of yoga, and rest in our essential nature, which is Oneness. This mantra doesn't mean to stop the fluctuations of the mind; especially at the beginning, the mind never stops. It's about observing the fluctuations and not identifying with them.

- *Aham Brahmasmi (Oneness):*

Translation: "I am the Universe."

In the most basic of terms, it is ones connection to the higherself or the Divine. It can also mean, "I am divine" or "I am sacred." We are all an embodiment of Source Energy, of the Divine, or if you will, God. Aham Brahmasmi is that acknowledgement that reflects in self and others.

- **Om Tat Sat (God)**

  Translation: "The Supreme Reality," or "All that is," or "Absolute truth."

  This mantra is thought to awaken our higher self and cultivate this higher consciousness so we can connect to the essence of who we really are. When partnered with the word, "Hari," it takes on a deeper of meaning of reminding us that we are more than the material and physical life. It takes on a life of not looking for reward but staying focused on what is good and true.

  This mantra instantly makes me think of the other mantra, "Yogastha Kuru Karmani," which is next.

- **Yogashta Kuru Karmani (Dharma then Karma):**

  Translation from the Bhagavad Gita, Chapter 2, Verse 48, translated by Eknath Easwaran: "Perform work in this world, Arjuna, as a man established within himself -without selfish attachments, and alike in success and defeat. For yoga is perfect evenness of mind."

  Dharma: "Right way of living," or "Path of rightness."

  Karma: A concept that ones action, deed, or work and the consequences that come from that action, deed, or work.

  This mantra is taking right action and putting good intention forward without worrying about the fruits the action(s) with bring about, as we are not entitled to the fruits.

- **Om Vasudhare Svaha (Buddhist Money Mantra):**

  Translation: "I pray to you, O Goddess Earth, bless me with abundance."

This mantra is chanted to attract wealth, prosperity and abundance in life. *Vasudhare* is the Earth Goddess, and her essential nature is abundance. Translated, her name means "stream of gems", which signifies the endless streams of prosperity that can flow into your life.

- *Om Zambala Zalendhraye Soha (Achieving Wealth):*

Translation: "You are the Lord of Valuable Treasures. Grant me the blessing of achieving wealth. Effortlessly, without desires. May all wishes be fulfilled."

In Buddhism, Zambala is known as the God of Wealth, and often perceived as the guard of money. Therefore, chanting this mantra is believed to attract wealth and prosperity, and to erradicate poverty.

- *Om Ami Dewa Hrih (Freedom from Illusion and Attachment):*

Translation: "Infinite, limitless light, illuminated Deity of Buddha nature with self-respect and dignity."

This mantra connects us to the Deity Amitabha, who is known as an embodiment of pure Light. As such, the mantra connects us with the Divine Light within, and frees us from illusions and attachment. The mantra can help to transcend limiting belief, and leads us to go beyond the mind, back to our perfect, Buddha-like nature.

- *Nam Myo Ho Renge Kyo (Fight Against Negativity):*

Translation is referencing The Lotus Sutra. "The ultimate Law or truth of the universe." This is according to the teachings of Nichiren.

This is a Japenese reading of Sanskrit and a Chinese phrase that is used to devote the mantra user to absolute truth and to align and even attach ones life with the eternal and unchanging truth. When you do this, it brings forth absolute and limitelss supply of wisdom for ones day to day life with all the changes.

- *Aham Vritti (Oneness):*

Translation: "I"-feeling or the "pure 'I am'-feeling," "I"-sense, or "I"-thought."

Beyond all thoughts, there is a background of stillness, pure beingness. Usually we identify with labels such as "I am a woman" or "I am happy." Aham Vritti brings us back to the pure I AM, to who we are beyond thought.

- *Yatha Pinde Tatha Brahmande (Cosmic/Human is One):*

Translation: "All that is outside you is within you."

This is a powerful, ancient mantra that reminds us that we has a human are a spark of Divine consciousness. Our self is part of the Self, the Cosmos, Divine Consciousness.

"Be still and know that I AM God." (Psalm 46:10)

BEAUTIFUL MANTRAS FOR ADVANCED PRACTITIONERS

For the advanced mantras, the space dedicated to them seems small into comparison of the layers and depth of meaning. These should be used with love, care, and understanding. I encourage you to look them up on YouTube and listen to their rhythmic sounds, if one resonates with you, then take it further by beginning a study. These mantras are rich in history and knowledge. The best way to embody these mantras is finding the one that resonates, then beginning your study of the mantra.

- *Tryambakam Mantra:* Om Try-Ambakam Yajaamahe, Sugandhim Pusstti-Vardhanam, Urvaarukam-Iva Bandhanaan, Mrtyor-Mukssiiya Maa-[A]mrtaat (Elimination of fear, calming of the soul, strength)

Translation: "Om, We Worship the Tryambaka (the Three-Eyed One), Who is Fragrant (as the Spiritual Essence), Increasing the Nourishment (of our Spiritual Core), From these many Bondages (of Samsara) similar to Cucumbers (tied to their Creepers), May I be Liberated from Death (Attachment to Perishable Things), So that I am not separated from the perception of Immortality (Immortal Essence pervading everywhere)."

This mantra is a verse from the Rig Veda 7.59.12 (ancient text) directed to Lord Shiva that is beneficial for mental, emotional, and physical health. People will also chant this mantra for others that are experiencing health obstacles.

- *Gayatri Mantra:* Om bhūr bhuvaḥ svaḥ, tát savitúr váreṇ(i)yam. bhárgo devásya dhīmahi, dhíyo yó naḥ prachodayat (Cleansing)

  Translation: "Om:the original sound; Bhur: the physical body/physical realm; Bhuvah: the life force/the mental realm Suvah: the soul/spiritual realm; Tat: That (God); Savitur: the Sun, Creator (source of all life); Vareñyam: adore; Bhargo: effulgence (divine light); Devasya: supreme Lord; Dheemahi: meditate; Dhiyo: the intellect; Yo: May this light; Nah: our; Prachodayāt: illumine/inspire."

  This mantra first appears in the Rig Veda, 03.62.10 and appears in later texts too. It is chanted for liberation, cleansing, it refines energy and connects to higher self.

- *Om Prabhu Deep Niranjan Saba Dukha Bhanjan (Oneness):*

  Meaning: "My adoration to the cosmic light, may my heart and entire being receive the divine light which purifies all my suffering, frees me from attachments and illumines my consciousness, may I merge and become one with the Universal Consciousness." - Yoga Daily Life

- *Tayata Om Bekanze Bekanze Maha Bekanze Radza Samudgate Soha (Remove Pain of Suffering):*

  Meaning: "May the many sentient beings who are sick, be freed from sickness soon. And may all the sicknesses of beings never arise again."

Just like in the last chapter, let's take some time to write down which mantras you would like to start with. Do not worry so much about proper pronunciation, it is the intention behind the mantra and accessing the vibration. Just like some people pronounce the word forest, as far-rest and others pronounce Boise as boy-zee instead of boy-see, we can get hung up where it really does not matter. Trust yourself, and let your heart guide you to the mantras that are calling you on this part of your journey.

_____

_____

_____

_____

_____

_____

_____

_____

_____

_____

_____

_____

_____

_____

_____

_____

_____

_____

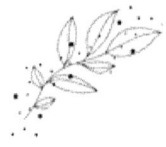

CONCLUSION
EMBRACING THE JOURNEY OF POSITIVE AFFIRMATIONS AND MANTRAS

As we reach the conclusion of this journey through "*The Art of Positive Affirmations and Mantras: Harnessing the Power for Personal Growth and Fulfillment,*" it's essential to reflect on the profound impact this practice can have on our lives. By now, you have immersed yourself in the transformative power of affirmations and mantras, understanding their ability to reshape your thoughts, emotions, and ultimately, your reality. This concluding chapter aims to encourage you to integrate this knowledge into your daily life and to revisit the teachings in this book whenever you need a refresher or a boost of inspiration.

Embracing Daily Practice: One of the key takeaways from this book is the importance of consistency in practicing affirmations and mantras. Just as physical exercise strengthens the body, mental and spiritual exercises strengthen the mind and soul. Make it a habit to start and end your day with positive affirmations. Choose mantras that resonate with your current goals and challenges. By doing so, you create a positive mental framework that influences your actions and decisions throughout the day.

Remember, the power of affirmations and mantras lies in their repetition and the belief you instill in them. Speak them with conviction, *feel* their truth, and let them guide your thoughts and actions. The more you practice, the more natural and effective they become.

Integrating Affirmations into Daily Life: Beyond dedicated sessions of affirmations and mantras, seek opportunities to integrate these practices into your everyday activities. Whether you are commuting, exercising, or performing routine tasks, use these moments to reinforce your positive statements. If you need help remembering your affirmations, use your notes in your phone or email them to yourself so they are accessible as the need arises. The mind is incredibly receptive to suggestions, especially during repetitive or mundane tasks. Utilize this time to embed empowering thoughts deeply into your subconscious.

Some examples would be: while driving to work, repeat affirmations about having a productive and fulfilling day. During exercise, focus on mantras that enhance your physical and mental strength. All of this creates a continuous flow of positive energy that supports your personal growth and fulfillment.

Revisiting the Teachings: Life is a dynamic journey with its ups and downs, and there will be times when you may feel disconnected from your practice or need a reminder of the principles you've learned. This book is designed to be a companion on your journey, a resource you can turn to whenever you need to change things up, find guidance or reinforcement.

Revisit the chapters that resonated with you the most. Reflect on the exercises that brought you clarity and empowerment. Allow the words within these pages to rekindle your motivation and strengthen your commitment to personal growth. Just as a good friend offers support and encouragement, let this book be your ally in times of need.

Embracing Community and Continuous Learning: Personal growth is not a solitary endeavor; it flourishes in the company of like-minded individuals. Seek out communities, both online and offline, where you can share your experiences and learn from others. Engaging with a supportive network can provide fresh perspectives, inspire new practices, and reinforce your commitment to positive affirmations and mantras.

The path of personal growth and fulfillment through positive affirmations and mantras is an ongoing journey, not a destination. Each step you take, each affirmation you speak, and each mantra you embrace brings you closer to a more empowered and enlightened version of yourself. Celebrate your progress, no matter how small, and be patient with yourself as you navigate this journey.

Remember, transformation takes time, and setbacks are a natural part of growth. When challenges arise, view them as opportunities to reaffirm your commitment to positive change.

Invitation to the Bonus Chapter: Before you go, we invite you to explore the bonus chapter. Here, you will find QR codes that lead to online resources, including affirmation and mantra videos, guided meditations, and support materials. These resources are designed to complement the teachings of this book and provide ongoing support as you continue your journey.

As you move forward, remember that the journey is just as important as the destination. Stay committed, stay positive, and let the wisdom of affirmations and mantras guide you toward a brighter, more empowered future.

Thank you for joining us on this journey and stay inspired on your path to personal growth and fulfillment!

B. M. Wolf

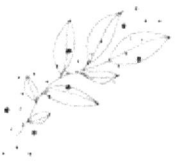

BONUS CHAPTER

Welcome to the bonus chapter, where you will find links and QR codes to resources and recordings! I just want to extend a very gracious thank you for trusting me to guide you through affirmations and mantras. A lot of love has gone into this book, and I hope you continue to explore by visiting the websites, social media, and recordings to help you along your journey. Follow me on IG @goldenalchemymeditation and TikTok @PeacePodBrandi.

AFFIRMATION RECORDINGS BY CATEGORY

Affirmations for Self-Love and Acceptance

Health and Well-Being

Success and Achievement

Wealth and Abundance

Gratitude and Appreciation

Relationships and Connection

Happiness and Joy

Spirituality and Inner Peace

Mantra Playlist

Nakshatra "Birthstar" Mantra

Wanderlust Malas and Reiki, Hand Tied, Reiki Infused, Mala Beads

https://www.wanderlustmalasandreiki.com/

Sign up for FREE Meditations

Meditations are delivered to your inbox monthly, along with exclusive offers and education.

Visit Golden Alchemy Meditation Website

Subscribe to my YouTube

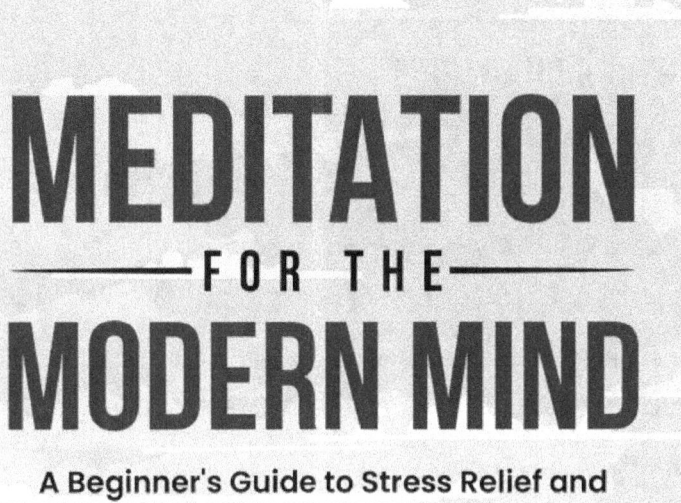

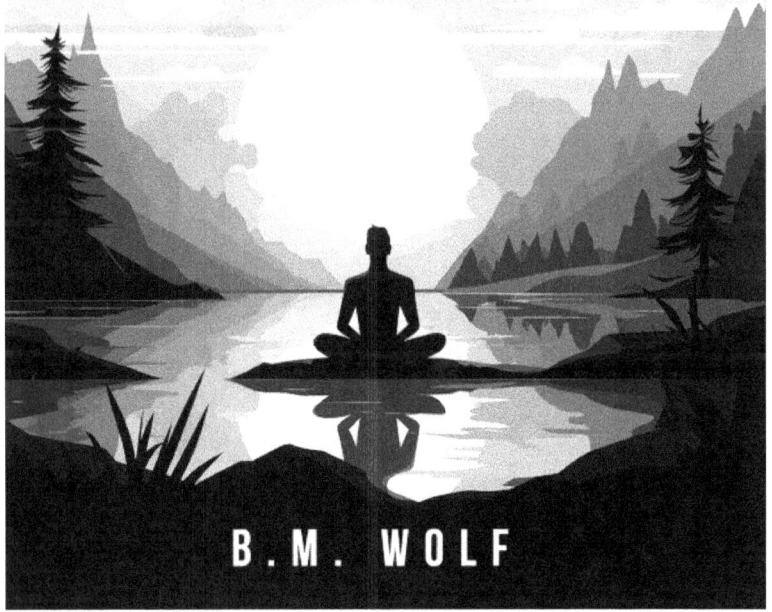

MEDITATION
— FOR THE —
MODERN MIND

A Beginner's Guide to Stress Relief and
Emotional Well-Being

B.M. WOLF

REFERENCES

REFERENCES CHAPTER 1

1. Old Dominion University. (n.d.). *Affirmations.*
   https://www.odu.edu/equity/civility-month/affirmations

2. Yoga Signs. (n.d.). *Difference between mantras and affirmations.*
   https://yogasigns.com/difference-between-mantras-and-affirmations/

3. Chopra, D. (n.d.). *What is a mantra.*
   https://chopra.com/blogs/meditation/what-is-a-mantra

4. Yogapedia. (n.d.). *Mantra.*
   https://www.yogapedia.com/definition/4950/mantra

5. Yogapedia. (n.d.). *Primordial sound mantra.*
   https://www.yogapedia.com/definition/10848/primordial-sound-mantra

6. Smart, L. (n.d.). *Your birthstar mantra.*
   https://lizsmart.com/your-birthstar-mantra

7. Kelly, S. M. (n.d.). Neuroplasticity and the power of your subconscious mind. LinkedIn.
   https://www.linkedin.com/pulse/neuroplasticity-power-your-subconscious-mind-sean-m-kelly

8. Schafer, J. (n.d.). How affirmations change your brain. LinkedIn.
   https://www.linkedin.com/pulse/how-affirmations-change-your-brain-jaeden-schafer-#:~:text=When%20you%20say%20an%20affirmation,to%20bring%20to%20your%20attention.

9. Sherman, K. J., Cherkin, D. C., Erro, J., Miglioretti, D. L., & Deyo, R. A. (2005). Comparing yoga, exercise, and a self-care book for chronic low back pain: A randomized, controlled trial. *Annals of Internal Medicine*, 143(12), 849–856.
    https://www.ncbi.nlm.nih.gov/pmc/articles/PMC4814782/

10. MentalHelp.net. (n.d.). *The science of affirmations*.
    https://www.mentalhelp.net/blogs/the-science-of-affirmations/

11. Sherman, K. J., Cherkin, D. C., Erro, J., Miglioretti, D. L., & Deyo, R. A. (2005). Comparing yoga, exercise, and a self-care book for chronic low back pain: A randomized, controlled trial. *Annals of Internal Medicine*, 143(12), 849–856.
    https://www.ncbi.nlm.nih.gov/pmc/articles/PMC4814782/

12. Stress Less, Live More. (n.d.). *The science of stress*.
    https://www.slma.cc/the-science-of-stress/

13. MD Anderson Cancer Center. (n.d.). *How stress affects cancer risk*.
    https://www.mdanderson.org/publications/focused-on-health/how-stress-affects-cancer-risk.h21-1589046.html

14. Zessin, U., Dickhäuser, O., & Garbade, S. (2015). The relationship between self-compassion and well-being: A meta-analysis. *Applied Psychology: Health and Well-Being*, 7(3), 340-364.
    https://www.ncbi.nlm.nih.gov/pmc/articles/PMC9623891/

15. Zessin, U., Dickhäuser, O., & Garbade, S. (2015). The relationship between self-compassion and well-being: A meta-analysis. *Applied Psychology: Health and Well-Being*, 7(3), 340-364.
    https://www.ncbi.nlm.nih.gov/pmc/articles/PMC9623891/

16. Zessin, U., Dickhäuser, O., & Garbade, S. (2015). The relationship between self-compassion and well-being: A meta-analysis. *Applied Psychology: Health and Well-Being*, 7(3), 340-364.
    https://www.ncbi.nlm.nih.gov/pmc/articles/PMC9623891/

REFERENCES CHAPTER 2

1. Bloomfully Paperie. (n.d.). Crafting positive affirmations: A guide to empowering your mindset.
   https://bloomfullypaperie.com/blogs/news/crafting-positive-affirmations-a-guide-to-empowering-your-mindset

2. MentalHelp.net. (n.d.). 140 daily chakra affirmations.
   https://www.mentalhelp.net/blogs/140-daily-chakra-affirmations/

3. Yoga International. (n.d.). What are the 7 chakras?.
   https://yogainternational.com/article/view/what-are-the-7-chakras/

REFERENCES CHAPTER 3

1. Pujayagna. (n.d.). What is mantra.
   https://pujayagna.com/blogs/facts-about-hinduism/what-is-mantra

2. Oxford Reference. (n.d.). Mantra.
   https://www.oxfordreference.com/display/10.1093/oi/authority.20110803100132631#:~:text=The%20word%20is%20Sanskrit%20and,Dictionary%20of%20Phrase%20and%20Fable%20»

3. Pujayagna. (n.d.). What is mantra.
   https://pujayagna.com/blogs/facts-about-hinduism/what-is-mantra

4. Ram Dass. (n.d.). How to use a mala.
   https://www.ramdass.org/use-mala/

5. Medium. (n.d.). How to practice japa meditation.
   https://medium.com/food-for-soul/how-to-practice-japa-meditation-1526fe6a7a5e

6. Himalayan Yoga Institute. (n.d.). What is so sacred about the number 108?.
   https://www.himalayanyogainstitute.com/what-is-so-sacred-about-the-number-108/

7. Ram Dass. (n.d.). How to use a mala.

https://www.ramdass.org/use-mala/

8. Medium. (n.d.). How to practice japa meditation. https://medium.com/food-for-soul/how-to-practice-japa-meditation-1526fe6a7a5e

9. Medium. (n.d.). How to practice japa meditation. https://medium.com/food-for-soul/how-to-practice-japa-meditation-1526fe6a7a5e

10. Hindu American Foundation. (n.d.). 5 things to know about Om. https://www.hinduamerican.org/blog/5-things-to-know-about-om

11. Ekhart Yoga. (n.d.). Everything changes on the mantra Aum. https://www.ekhartyoga.com/articles/practice/everything-changes-on-the-mantra-aum

12. Ananda. (n.d.). Aum. https://www.ananda.org/yogapedia/aum/

13. Mindbodygreen. (n.d.). What does the Om symbol mean. https://www.mindbodygreen.com/articles/what-does-the-om-symbol-mean

14. Islam, Md. J., & Ahmad, Md. M. (2009). Development of a new wireless ad-hoc network for communication among electronic devices. *International Journal of Computer Science and Network Security, 9*(1), 295-301. http://paper.ijcsns.org/07_book/200901/20090151.pdf

15. Mindbodygreen. (n.d.). What does the Om symbol mean. https://www.mindbodygreen.com/articles/what-does-the-om-symbol-mean

16. Sadhana Yoga. (n.d.). Your guide to beginning a mantra practice. https://sadhanayoga.com/your-guide-to-beginning-a-mantra-practice/

17. Sadhana Yoga. (n.d.). Your guide to beginning a mantra practice. https://sadhanayoga.com/your-guide-to-beginning-a-mantra-practice/

18. Jindal, V., Gupta, S., Das, R., & Jindal, A. (2013). Clinical practice of yoga: Meditation and mantra. *International Journal of Yoga, 6*(2), 139–141.

19. Dusek, J. A., Otu, H. H., Wohlhueter, A. L., Bhasin, M., Zerbini, L. F., Joseph, M. G., ... Libermann, T. A. (2008). Genomic counter-stress changes induced by the relaxation response. *PLOS ONE, 3*(7), e2576.

20. Goldin, P. R., & Gross, J. J. (2010). Effects of mindfulness-based stress reduction (MBSR) on emotion regulation in social anxiety disorder. *Emotion, 10*(1), 83–91.

21. Deep Ho'oponopono. (n.d.). A concise history of Ho'oponopono. https://deephooponopono.com/a-concise-history-of-hooponopono/

REFERENCES CHAPTER 4

1. Brain & Behavior Research Foundation. (n.d.). Self-love and what it means. https://bbrfoundation.org/blog/self-love-and-what-it-means#:~:text=Self%2Dlove%20is%20a%20state,well%2Dbeing%20to%20please%20others.

2. Brain & Behavior Research Foundation. (n.d.). Self-love and what it means. https://bbrfoundation.org/blog/self-love-and-what-it-means#:~:text=Self%2Dlove%20is%20a%20state,well%2Dbeing%20to%20please%20others.

3. HeartMath Institute. (n.d.). Personal heart coherence. https://www.heartmath.org/heart-coherence/personal/

4. Braden, G. (n.d.). Resilience from the heart. https://greggbraden.com/resilience-from-the-heart/

5. Tolle, E. (1997). *The power of now.* New World Library.

6. Forbes Coaches Council. (2021, May 6). Four brain science habits to help neutralize negative self-talk. https://www.forbes.com/sites/forbescoachescouncil/2021/05/06/four-brain-science-habits-to-help-neutralize-negative-self-talk/?sh=eed09194f3ca

7. VanderWeele, T. J., & Rodriguez, L. (2019). Meditation and health: An updated meta-analysis. *Journal of Alternative and Complementary Medicine, 25*(11), 1165-1170.

8. PubMed Central. (2021). The impact of mindfulness meditation on mental health. *Mindfulness, 12*(3), 506-520.

9. Castrillon, C. (2020, July 12). 5 ways to go from a scarcity to abundance mindset. Forbes. https://www.forbes.com/sites/carolinecastrillon/2020/07/12/5-ways-to-go-from-a-scarcity-to-abundance-mindset/?sh=18b6d9641197

10. Bright Inventions. (n.d.). How to develop a solution-oriented mindset in your life and in your team. https://brightinventions.pl/blog/how-to-develop-solution-oriented-mindset-in-your-life-and-in-your-team/

REFERENCES CHAPTER 5

1. Perry, G. (n.d.). Mantra around the world. Gemma Perry. https://www.gemmaperryom.com/post/mantra-arond-the-world

2. Perry, G. (n.d.). Mantra around the world. Gemma Perry. https://www.gemmaperryom.com/post/mantra-arond-the-world

3. Sound of Life. (n.d.). Sounding off on spirituality: Exploring chanting in different cultures. https://www.soundoflife.com/blogs/places/sounding-off-on-spirituality-exploring-chanting-different-cultures

4. PubMed Central. (2010). Mantra and mental health benefits. *Journal of Mental Health and Clinical Psychology, 14*(2), 45-58.

https://www.ncbi.nlm.nih.gov/pmc/articles/PMC2952121/

5. Verywell Mind. (2021). Mantras: Mental health benefits. https://www.verywellmind.com/mantras-mental-health-benefits-7112640

6. Wanderlust Mala & Reiki. (n.d.). About Wanderlust Mala & Reiki. https://www.wanderlustmalasandreiki.com/about

7. Sathya Sai International Organization. (n.d.). Gayatri mantra. https://www.sathyasai.org/devotional/gayatri

8. Yoga International. (n.d.). The Gayatri mantra: Awakening to the sun. https://yogainternational.com/article/view/the-gayatri-mantra-awakening-to-the-sun/

9. Meditative Mind. (n.d.). Om Hum mantra: Benefits and meaning. https://meditativemind.org/om-hum-mantra-benefits-meaning/

10. Japa Mala Beads. (n.d.). So Hum mantra. https://japamalabeads.com/so-hum-mantra/

11. Mindworks. (n.d.). What is mantra meditation?. https://mindworks.org/blog/what-is-mantra-meditation/

12. 3HO Foundation. (n.d.). Kirtan Kriya meditation. https://www.3ho.org/meditation/kirtan-kriya/

13. Alzheimer's Research & Prevention Foundation. (n.d.). Research on Kirtan Kriya yoga exercise. https://alzheimersprevention.org/research/kirtan-kriya-yoga-exercise/

14. 3HO Foundation. (n.d.). Kirtan Kriya meditation. https://www.3ho.org/meditation/kirtan-kriya/

15. 3HO Foundation. (n.d.). Kirtan Kriya meditation. https://www.3ho.org/meditation/kirtan-kriya/

16. 3HO Foundation. (n.d.). Kirtan Kriya meditation. https://www.3ho.org/meditation/kirtan-kriya/

17. 3HO Foundation. (n.d.). Kirtan Kriya meditation.
https://www.3ho.org/meditation/kirtan-kriya/

18. Foundation for the Preservation of the Mahayana Tradition (FPMT). (n.d.). The benefits of chanting Om Mani Padme Hum.
https://fpmt.org/education/teachings/lama-zopa-rinpoche/the-benefits-of-chanting-om-mani-padme-hum/

19. Buddha Groove. (n.d.). Om Mani Padme Hum.
https://blog.buddhagroove.com/om-mani-padme-hum/

20. Foundation for the Preservation of the Mahayana Tradition (FPMT). (n.d.). The benefits of chanting Om Mani Padme Hum.
https://fpmt.org/education/teachings/lama-zopa-rinpoche/the-benefits-of-chanting-om-mani-padme-hum/

21. Foundation for the Preservation of the Mahayana Tradition (FPMT). (n.d.). The benefits of chanting Om Mani Padme Hum.
https://fpmt.org/education/teachings/lama-zopa-rinpoche/the-benefits-of-chanting-om-mani-padme-hum/

REFERENCES CHAPTER 6

1. Window Still. (n.d.). The science of manifestation: How visualization can help you create your own reality.
https://www.windowstill.com/the-science-of-manifestation-how-visualization-can-help-you-create-your-own-reality/posts/

2. Window Still. (n.d.). The science of manifestation: How visualization can help you create your own reality.
https://www.windowstill.com/the-science-of-manifestation-how-visualization-can-help-you-create-your-own-reality/posts/

3. PubMed. (2009). Study on the science of intention. *Journal of Psychology, 123*(2), 45-56.
https://pubmed.ncbi.nlm.nih.gov/19245175/

4. PubMed. (2009). Study on the science of intention. *Journal of Psychology, 123*(2), 45-56.
https://pubmed.ncbi.nlm.nih.gov/19245175/

5. Institute of Noetic Sciences. (n.d.). Three remarkable studies on the science of intention.
https://noetic.org/blog/three-remarkable-studies-on-the-science-of-intention/

REFERENCES CHAPTER 7

1. Hay, L. (n.d.). What is mirror work?.
https://www.louisehay.com/what-is-mirror-work/

2. Hay, L. (n.d.). What is mirror work?.
https://www.louisehay.com/what-is-mirror-work/

REFERENCES CHAPTER 8

1. Chopra, D. (n.d.). 9 powerful mantras in Sanskrit and Gurmukhi.
https://chopra.com/blogs/personal-growth/9-powerful-mantras-in-sanskrit-and-gurmukhi

2. Temple Purohit. (n.d.). List of powerful mantras: Significance & benefits.
https://www.templepurohit.com/list-powerful-mantras-significance-benefits/

3. Davidji. (n.d.). Yoga, Chitta Vritti Nirodha & radiating strength.
https://davidji.com/yoga-chitta-vritti-nirodha-radiating-strength/

4. Times of India. (n.d.). 6 mantras that can help you transform your life.
https://timesofindia.indiatimes.com/life-style/soul-search/6-mantras-that-can-help-you-transform-your-life/photostory/106300120.cms

5. Level. (n.d.). 9 Buddhist mantras that will radically improve your life.
https://level.game/blogs/9-buddhist-mantras-that-will-radically-improve-your-life?lang=en

6. Greenmesg. (n.d.). Mahamrityunjaya Mantra: Lord Shiva's mantra for healing.
    https://greenmesg.org/stotras/shiva/mahamrityunjaya_mantra.php

7. Wildmind. (n.d.). Mantras for meditation.
    https://www.wildmind.org/mantras/

8. Yogapedia. (n.d.). Yogapedia.
    https://www.yogapedia.com/

9. Sat Nam. (n.d.). Sat Nam Rasayan.
    https://www.satnam.de/de/sat-nam-rasayan-guru-dev-singh.html

10. Kirbanu. (n.d.). Om Vasudhare Svaha.
    https://kirbanu.com/om-vasudhare-svaha/

11. Mandalas Life. (2018). The Zambala Money Guard.
    https://mandalas.life/2018/the-zambala-money-guard/

12. Dto Music. (n.d.). Om Ami Dewa Hrih.
    https://dtomusic.com/om-ami-dewa-hrih/

13. Yogapedia. (n.d.). Om Tat Sat.
    https://www.yogapedia.com/definition/6623/om-tat-sat

14. Nichiren Library. (n.d.). Nichiren Library.
    https://www.nichirenlibrary.org/en/dic/Content/N/11

15. Greenmesg. (n.d.). Mahamrityunjaya Mantra: Lord Shiva's mantra for healing.
    https://greenmesg.org/stotras/shiva/mahamrityunjaya_mantra.php

16. Shlokam. (n.d.). Tryambakam mantra.
    https://shlokam.org/tryambakam/

17. Dragonfly Yoga. (n.d.). Ten yoga mudras and their benefits.
    https://www.dragonfly-yoga.org/blog/ten-yoga-mudras-and-their-benefits-1

18. Ekhart Yoga. (n.d.). An introduction to mudras.

https://www.ekhartyoga.com/articles/practice/an-introduction-to-mudras

19. https://www.sathyasai.org/devotional/gayatri

20. https://brisbane.yogaindailylife.org.au/blog/2015/12/22/mantra---what-to-repeat-as-a-source-of-power-and-achievement1

21. https://chopra.com/blogs/personal-growth/9-powerful-mantras-in-sanskrit-and-gurmukhi